T028614

W5418

KT-548-157

OF01032

Books should be returned to the SDH Library on or before
the date stamped above unless a renewal has been arranged

Salisbury District Hospital Library

Telephone: Salisbury (01722) 336262 extn. 4432 / 33

Out of hours answer machine in operation

Occupational Therapy Models for Intervention with Children and Families

Occupational Therapy Models for Intervention with Children and Families

Sandra Barker Dunbar, DPA, OTR/L
Chair and Professor
Occupational Therapy Department
Nova Southeastern University
Fort Lauderdale, Florida

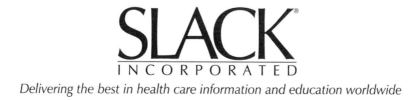

Delivering the best in health care information and education worldwide

www.slackbooks.com

ISBN: 978-1-55642-763-3

Occupational Therapy Models for Intervention with Children and Families, Instructor's Manual, is also available from SLACK Incorporated. Don't miss this important companion to this book. To obtain the *Instructor's Manual,* please visit www.efacultylounge.com.

The procedures and practices described in this book should be implemented in a manner consistent with the professional standards set for the circumstances that apply in each specific situation. Every effort has been made to confirm the accuracy of the information presented and to correctly relate generally accepted practices. The authors, editor, and publisher cannot accept responsibility for errors or exclusions or for the outcome of the material presented herein. There is no expressed or implied warranty of this book or information imparted by it. Care has been taken to ensure that drug selection and dosages are in accordance with currently accepted/recommended practice. Due to continuing research, changes in government policy and regulations, and various effects of drug reactions and interactions, it is recommended that the reader carefully review all materials and literature provided for each drug, especially those that are new or not frequently used. Any review or mention of specific companies or products is not intended as an endorsement by the author or publisher.

SLACK Incorporated uses a review process to evaluate submitted material. Prior to publication, educators or clinicians provide important feedback on the content that we publish. We welcome feedback on this work.

Published by: SLACK Incorporated
                       6900 Grove Road
                       Thorofare, NJ 08086 USA
                       Telephone: 856-848-1000
                       Fax: 856-853-5991
                       www.slackbooks.com

Contact SLACK Incorporated for more information about other books in this field or about the availability of our books from distributors outside the United States.

Library of Congress Cataloging-in-Publication Data

Dunbar, Sandra Barker
  Occupational therapy models for intervention with children and families / Sandra Barker Dunbar.
     p. ; cm.
  Includes bibliographical references and index.
  ISBN 978-1-55642-763-3 (alk. paper)
1. Occupational therapy for children. 2. Occupational therapy services. I. Dunbar, Sandra Barker [DNLM:
  1. Occupational Therapy--methods. 2. Child. 3. Family. WS 368 O156 2007]

RJ53.O25O235 2007
618.92'89165--dc22

                              2007001927

Printed in the United States of America.

Last digit is print number: 10   9   8   7   6   5   4   3   2

Dedication

Dedicated to the memory of my mother, Matilda (Syd) Nowell Barker, PhD, and my son, Jaden.

Contents

Acknowledgments

Many thanks to all of the occupational therapists, occupational scientists, and occupational therapy students for their contributions to this text. Thanks also to the numerous families who permitted their stories to be told in the form of case examples throughout the chapters.

About the Author

Sandra (Sandee) Barker Dunbar, DPA, OTR/L, has practiced occupational therapy with children and families for more than 20 years. She received her Bachelor of Science degree in Occupational Therapy from Loma Linda University, her Master of Arts degree in Occupational Therapy from New York University, and her Doctor of Public Administration degree from Nova Southeastern University.

Sandee's initial occupational therapy work was in early intervention, neonatal intensive care, and community-based intervention. Sandee has enjoyed developing a variety of innovative programs for families, including a primary care approach to early identification of developmental issues in collaboration with a pediatrician, Dr. Rose Joseph.

Currently, Sandee is Chair and Professor in the Occupational Therapy Program at Nova Southeastern University. Since 1995, Sandee has contributed to student learning at NSU while maintaining a link to clinical and community settings that are geared toward helping children and families. This includes supervising students in on-campus pre-service learning at the Baudhuin School of the Mailman Segal Institute, which serves hundreds of children with autism each year.

Sandee continues to be committed to creatively finding ways to better meet family needs for children with and without disabilities. She is grateful for the support of family, co-workers, and friends for their shared vision of making life better for those in need.

Contributing Authors

Erna Imperatore Blanche, PhD, OTR/L, FAOTA
Associate Professor of Clinical Practice
Department of Occupational Science and
Therapy
University of Southern California
Co-Director Therapy West
Los Angeles, California

Patricia Bowyer, EdD, OTR/L, BCN
Post-Doctoral Research Associate
University of Illinois at Chicago
Chicago, Illinois

Beth Werner DeGrace, PhD, OTR/L
Assistant Professor
Department of Rehabilitation Science
College of Allied Health
University of Oklahoma Health Sciences
Center
Oklahoma City, Oklahoma

Winnie Dunn, PhD, OTR, FAOTA
Professor and Chair
Department of Occupational Therapy
Education
School of Allied Health
University of Kansas Medical Center
Kansas City, Kansas

Dominique Blanche Kiefer, OTD, OTR/L
Independent Contractor
Philadelphia, Pennsylvania

Jessica M. Kramer, MS, OTR/L
Head Research Assistant MOHO
Clearinghouse
PhD Student, Disability Studies
University of Illinois at Chicago
Chicago, Illinois

Mary Law, PhD, OT(C)
Professor and Associate Dean (Health
Sciences) Rehabilitation Science
Co-Director, CanChild Centre for
Childhood Disability Research
McMaster University
Hamilton, Ontario, Canada

Christine Teeters Myers, MHS, OTR/L
Visiting Assistant Professor
Department of Occupational Therapy
Eastern Kentucky University
Richmond, Kentucky

Shirley O'Brien, MS, OTR/L, FAOTA
Associate Professor
Department of Occupational Therapy
Eastern Kentucky University
Richmond, Kentucky

Doris Pierce, PhD, OTR/L, FAOTA
Endowed Chair in Occupational Therapy
Eastern Kentucky University
Richmond, Kentucky

Mary Ellen Thompson, MS, OTR/L
Assistant Professor
Department of Occupational Therapy
Midwestern University
Glendale, Arizona

Foreword

In the mid-1960s, Mary Reilly proposed that the uniqueness of occupational therapy should be its emphasis on occupation and that engagement in meaningful occupation was the key to recovery from illness. In the classic statement from her Eleanor Clark Slagle address, "Man, through the use of his hands, as they are energized by mind and will, can influence the state of his own health" (Reilly, 1962, p. 2), she urged the profession to return to the founding principle of occupational therapy, that being a balance of work, play, and rest. She described "a theory, specific for occupational therapy, which proposes the play-work continuum called occupational behavior as the theoretical framework for practice and education" (Reilly, 1969, p. 299). She further designed the curriculum at the University of Southern California around occupational behavior, and many of her students researched various aspects of occupational behavior.

Over the years, former students of Dr. Reilly and others embraced and further refined the concepts of occupation and purposeful activity as frames within which to evaluate and treat clients, and they developed other models of practice. In 2002, the American Occupational Therapy Association firmly positioned occupation as the core of our practice with the adoption of the *Occupational Therapy Practice Framework*. In addition, the current demands of health care, the legislative initiatives, and the expansion of occupational therapy into nontraditional areas of practice have emphasized the need for holistic models to guide clinical reasoning and treatment of children and their families.

With this background, it is exciting to read this book which compiles the most recent and most utilized models of practice for occupational therapists dealing with children, youth, and their families and to see that all these models view children as occupational beings within the context of their families and society.

The first chapter defines and differentiates between theory, frame of reference, and model and puts the models into perspective within the demands of society today. Subsequent chapters describe the models and their development, describe assessment tools and intervention methods, and apply the models through extensive case studies. Chapter 2 utilizes occupational science as a context within which to apply the frames of reference of Sensory Integration and Neurodevelopmental Treatment. The concept of Lifestyle Redesign is applied to address the family and lifestyle issues of children with sensory integrative or neurodevelopmental problems. In Chapter 3, the Person-Environment-Occupation model is used to analyze factors influencing the occupational performance of children and youth. The model uses a family-centered approach to identify barriers and strengths and guide intervention. Chapter 4 describes the Model of Human Occupation and applies its concepts to evaluation, intervention, and outcome. Literature is presented that supports evidence-based application of the model.

Chapter 5 discusses the Occupational Adaptation model and describes the person, the occupational environment, and the interaction among these to afford occupation. It describes occupational challenges and the process of adaptation, as well as the therapist's role as facilitator. In Chapter 6, Ecology of Human Performance model, the constructs of person, context, task, and performance are discussed and the model is used to structure interdisciplinary practice serving children and their families.

Chapter 7 synthesizes all these models, describes the clinical reasoning process that therapists use to support occupation-based family-centered practice and proposes the process of Occupation by Design for decision making. This approach targets the therapeutic intervention and judges it on appeal, contextual intactness, and accuracy. The unique contributions that each of the models provide are discussed from this process and a longitudinal case is used to illustrate how these models can be integrated.

All the models focus on occupation, are client/family centered, are contextualized, and are in concert with the *Practice Framework*. They all emphasize the clinical reasoning process in which therapists engage when treating clients. Most importantly, they all reinforce occupational therapy's domain of concern and illustrate the profession's unique expertise in providing service to children and their families. This should be an essential text for occupational therapy curricula, practitioners, and researchers.

Susan H. Knox, PhD, OTR/L, FAOTA
Director Emerita
Therapy in Action
Tarzana, California

References

American Occupational Therapy Association. (2002). Occupational therapy practice framework: Domain and process. *American Journal of Occupational Therapy, 56*, 609-639.

Reilly, M. (1962). Occupational therapy can be one of the great ideas of 20th century medicine. *American Journal of Occupational Therapy, 16*(1), 1-9.

Reilly, M. (1969). The educational process. *American Journal of Occupational Therapy, 23*(4), 299-307.

Introduction

Occupational therapists have a long history of working with children, including services for individuals with deafness and blindness in the 1950s, to the expansion of school-based practice in the 1970s, to early intervention practice in the 1980s. Currently, there are endless opportunities for impacting participation in childhood occupations, as well as ensuring that family occupational needs are met in the variety of practice settings in which we work.

The challenge continues, however, to practice in a way that family-centered care mandates are truly being met and that the family is the central consideration in practice. We continue to struggle with our ideals as "experts" and may unknowingly limit ourselves, as well as the families we interface with, by neglecting to address the whole person and the whole family unit.

The challenge also includes a need to consistently view children through an occupational lens, rather than limiting ourselves to a component orientation. There is a need to see classroom participation, rather than just pencil grip; to see peer interaction, rather than just attention span; to see successful involvement in a physical education class, rather than just trunk rotation; to see mother-infant interaction, rather than just a sucking pattern. The use of a wider lens for evaluation and intervention will enable us to better meet the occupational needs of children.

It is the particular challenges of providing authentic family-centered and occupation-centered services that led to consideration of a text that would address ways to view occupational therapy practice with children and families in a different way. Traditional frames of reference offer significant strategies for impacting specific areas of practice. They have served occupational therapists well in that they provide methods of evaluation, distinctions of what is function and what is dysfunction, as well as treatment strategies to optimize functioning for specific skill areas. However, there remains a need for integrating these aspects into a broader schema, such as a model, for optimal provision of occupation-centered services. Chapter 1 elaborates on these aspects and provides a distinction between a frame of reference and a model that will enable comparative analysis as the reader reviews the subsequent chapters.

The discipline of occupational science provides an avenue for facilitating awareness and understanding of the significance of occupations. This creates a bridge for then understanding children and families, their ways of being, and how they construct their daily routines. Chapter 2 provides an overview of how occupational science considerations can be related to practice with children who may have developmental issues.

The text does not provide an all-inclusive approach to models for practice with children and families. There are numerous models that one may consider that are not mentioned in this format. The reader is encouraged to explore alternate models and compare them to the ones in the text to assess what is the best fit for his or her current (or future) practice and philosophical viewpoints. The Person-Environment-Occupation model, the Model of Human Occupation, the Occupational Adaptation model, and the Ecology of Human Performance model are addressed in this sequence following Chapter 2. Each chapter is written by either the model author or recognized colleagues of the author. The culminating chapter provides an overview and integrative approach utilizing Occupation by Design.

The numerous cases and learning activities throughout each chapter are intended to facilitate much processing and discussion. The accompanying *Instructor's Manual* provides further learning activities that will assist the instructor in elaborating on the chapter highlights and providing classroom experiences that will enhance student learning.

Occupational therapists have the privilege of impacting countless children and families. It is hoped that this information will further enhance our ability to optimally meet the growing occupational needs of our clients in the myriad of arenas where we work and play.

Sandra Barker Dunbar, DPA, OTR/L
Chair and Professor
Occupational Therapy Department
Nova Southeastern University
Fort Lauderdale, Florida

THEORY, FRAME OF REFERENCE, AND MODEL: A DIFFERENTIATION FOR PRACTICE CONSIDERATIONS

Sandra Barker Dunbar, DPA, OTR/L

Learning Objectives

At the end of this chapter, the reader will be able to:
- Define a theory, frame of reference, and model.
- Identify the differences between a theory, frame of reference, and model.
- Identify theories that have contributed to occupational therapy frames of reference and models.
- Understand current practice issues that create opportunities for intervention from a model perspective.

The early development of the occupational therapy profession was impacted by various philosophies, such as humanism and pragmatism. The initial formation of the profession occurred within the context of a broader societal movement to better serve those in need. During the early 20th century, negative effects of industrialization, increasing public awareness of inhumane treatment for the mentally ill, and growing problems related to urban living, provided a need for improvements in societal conditions (Peloquin, 2000). Physicians, nurses, philosophers, social workers, and others worked together to create a more humane approach to addressing societal needs.

Humanistic philosophy incorporates the belief that people are capable of ethical conduct, as well as finding ways for self-fulfillment (Herrick, 2005). Pragmatism includes the belief that meaning may be determined by practical consequences (Ayer, 2005). These philosophies, as well as others, enabled early pioneers in occupational therapy to foster beliefs regarding the benefits of occupation and an individual's need to participate in meaningful activity (Peloquin, 2000).

Although the philosophies of the early years in the profession helped to guide occupational therapists in their selection of treatment activities, there were no occupational therapy models or frames of reference that delineated specific treatment guidelines for the growing areas of practice. During the 1960s, this began to change with the emergence of theoretical frameworks such as Mary Reilly's Occupational Behavior (Reilly, 1966). Reilly believed that there is an inherent need to engage in occupation and that through occupation, individuals can master their environment. In addition, the developmental continuum of play and work contributes to the ability to become competent and be successful in occupational roles (Reilly, 1969). This shift to a more formalized theoretical foundation provided occupational therapy an increasingly valid status as a profession.

Throughout the occupational therapy literature there are numerous definitions and descriptions of theories, frames of reference, and models. The inconsistencies in the literature have led professionals to use terms interchangeably and with uncertainty when discussing theories, frames of reference, and models. Establishing a more consistent language throughout the profession will enhance practitioners' ability to participate in professional dialogue in a more effective manner.

In order to understand models for practice with children and their families in this particular text, it is critical to differentiate a theory and frame of reference from a model. The reader will better understand the intent of focusing on models for this work when the differentiation is clarified and consistent throughout.

Anne Mosey's efforts at constructing a solid foundation for deciphering what a profession is and how occupational therapy is a profession enlightened occupational therapists in a significant way. Her work offers consistent definitions and descriptions that are critical for understanding the differences between a theory, frame of reference, and model (Mosey, 1981, 1996). These definitions and descriptions will be the rubric for the differentiation in this text due to the consistency in Mosey's work and the alignment with theoretical literature external to the occupational therapy profession. Authors who have more recently identified similar distinctions include Kramer, Hinojosa, and Royeen (2003); Baum and Christiansen (2005); as well as Braveman and Kielhofner (2006). Their descriptions will also be incorporated into some of the subsequent overviews.

Theory

The characteristics of a profession include the derivation of material from science and learning. This scientific inquiry leads to theory development that can provide a means for identifying and expressing key ideas within an area of practice (Walker & Avant, 1995). Descriptions and explanations regarding relationships between people, health, environment, and other factors enable practitioners to understand the complexity of occupation and optimal participation in daily life. Academic disciplines such as sociology, psychology, and anthropology have all contributed theories that describe relationships between occupation and health (Nelson & Jepson-Thomas, 2003). Theories form the basis of occupational therapy frames of reference and models, as well as paradigms that provide specific knowledge about perspective in the occupational therapy profession (Braveman & Kielhofner, 2006).

Mosey defines *theory* as "an abstract description of a circumscribed set of observable events" (1981, p. 30). A theory provides explanations regarding how certain situations occur and how events are related. The intended purpose of a theory is to predict the relationship between the particular events (Mosey, 1981).

In occupational therapy practice with children and families, therapists rely on many theories to understand the relationship between events. Occupational therapy students are exposed to a variety of human development theories in prerequisite education or in occupational therapy curricula. This exposure enables the occupational therapist to understand the foundation for many occupational therapy frames of reference that are often applied to practice with children.

Table 1-1
PIAGET'S STAGES OF COGNITIVE DEVELOPMENT

Stages of Cognition	*Description*
Sensorimotor Period 0 to 2 years	A progression from reflex-dominated activity to mental representation of objects that leads to cognitively combining and manipulating items in play. This stage is dominated by practice play.
Preoperational Thought Period 2 to 7 years	First level of stage to 4 years is characterized by dependence on perception, rather than on logic for problem solving. Egocentric speech is present. The second level of the stage is characterized by a transition to dependence on logical thought for problem solving. Symbolic play to sociodramatic play is observed during this stage.
Concrete Operations Period 7 to 11 years	Performance of logical mental operations on observed or imagined objects. Games with rules are common during this stage as the child assimilates to social demands.
Formal Operations Period 11 to 15 years	Imagination of past, present, and future conditions that will influence a situation. Logic used to hypothesize multiple ways of solving a problem.

A well-known human development theory is Piaget's Cognitive Development theory (Piaget, 1950). Piaget's work is also often referred to as a theory of cognitive development. This theory will be used to illustrate the intent of theory, as well as to be applied to occupational therapy practice with children. Piaget, a renowned Swiss developmental psychologist, presented mental growth as advancing through four main levels. These levels (Table 1-1) include sensorimotor (0 to 2 years), preoperational thought (2 to 7 years), concrete operations (7 to 11 years), and formal operations (11 to 15 years). Beyond the midteen years, cognitive processes move away from an egocentric standpoint to a view that encompasses influences from society and the realities of everyday living in context with associations with others. Although the theory has been critiqued as not being sensitive to a wide variety of cultures and individuals from varying socioeconomic groups, it continues to be widely referred to and applied (Thomas, 1999).

The predictive nature of a theory allows one to foretell or anticipate what will occur under certain circumstances. Piaget's Cognitive Development theory provides sequential stages that a child will typically move through given adequate environmental supports for development of the cognitive processes. In addition, a theory will establish relationships between events and circumstances. Piaget was considered an interactionist who credited heredity and environment with a combined impact on child development (Thomas, 1999).

By this example, occupational therapists can relate to the significance of theory on practice. The relationship of environmental supports to cognitive development is critical in the understanding of child development and subsequent treatment planning for children with compromised occupational performance. In addition, the predictive value of stage-related functioning can assist occupational therapists in understanding what skills will develop next in specific areas of functioning, including object and social play.

A specific example of how Piaget's theory has influenced occupational therapy in practice with children is noted in Hurff's Competency Model (Hurff, 1980). Hurff describes a play skills inventory as a means of establishing competency in a 10-year-old child. A pyramid figure in the article depicts a hierarchy of competency skills that mirrors Piaget's cognitive development stages. In Hurff's work, the lower stage is termed "Sensation Motor" and consists of input from the various senses, as well as gross motor experiences. In the second stage, "Perception," Hurff describes personal control, role learning, conceptualization, and social perception as key characteristics of this developmental stage. At the top of the pyramid, the child achieves a level of "Intellect" that is characterized by reasoning, thinking, problem solving, and learning (Hurff, 1980). Clearly, this is comparable to Piaget's stages of cognitive development. The influence of Piaget's work in occupational therapy is notable and enables occupational therapists to understand the significance of theory in connection to practice.

Frame of Reference

Mosey defines a *frame of reference* as "a set of interrelated internally consistent concepts, definitions, and postulates that provide a systematic description of and prescription for a practitioner's interaction within a particular aspect of a profession's domain of concern" (Mosey, 1981, p. 129). A frame of reference delineates a specific area of practice and provides consistent language in order to support intervention for a particular aspect.

Criteria for a frame of reference are consistent throughout Mosey's writings (Mosey, 1970, 1981, 1996) and are based on other professional literature that highlights the particulars of a profession vs. a discipline (Ford & Urban, 1963; Friedson; 1970).

A frame of reference consists of four primary aspects, including a theoretical base, function-dysfunction continuums, descriptions of behaviors that are indicative of function and dysfunction, and postulates regarding change (Mosey, 1981).

A theoretical base provides a foundation for a frame of reference by delineating specific concepts and their definitions. For instance, the Neurodevelopmental Treatment (NDT) frame of reference that is widely used in practice with children is founded on human developmental and neurodevelopmental theories (Bobath, 1971). These form the basis for understanding the delineated area of practice and support the selection of appropriate treatment activities that fall within the parameters of the frame of reference. Developmental concepts are consistent and serve as a guide to evaluation and treatment for children, as well as adults with neuromotor-oriented dysfunction (Schoen & Anderson, 1999).

The function-dysfunction continuum is a range description of one area related to human performance (Mosey, 1996). The range describes complete ability in a particular skill to an inability to demonstrate the same skill. For instance, considering NDT again, the following example of a function-dysfunction continuum illustrates the degree of range for a particular skill expected to be observed within the parameters of this frame of reference.

Inability to crawl to retrieve a toy ⟵⟶ Ability to crawl to retrieve a toy

The continuum aspect indicates that there is an ongoing therapeutic endeavor for the client to move within the range to attain the goal of a demonstrated skill or participation in a particular activity.

The behavioral descriptions of function and dysfunction are critical for understanding the range and what is expected at different levels of performance. This enables an occupational therapist to identify what is function and what is dysfunction within the delineated area of concern. Behaviors indicative of function within NDT include age-appropriate mobility, the use of automatic responses for the maintenance of functional balance, and varied movements to meet the demands of the environment. Examples of behaviors indicative of dysfunction within this frame of reference include a persistence of primitive reflex activity, contractures, or a predominance of certain postures that can interfere with function (Schoen & Anderson, 1999). Identifying behaviors of function and dysfunction is part of the evaluation and ongoing reassessment process within any frame of reference. The primary means of evaluation within the NDT frame of reference is observation. However, other frames of reference, such as Sensory Integration ([SI] which is also recognized as a theory), provide extensive and well-founded methods for identifying function and dysfunction (Ayres, 1989).

The last aspect of a frame of reference is the postulates regarding change. These are prescriptive statements, based on the theoretical base, that identify strategies to address the dysfunction through therapeutic intervention. The statements include the detail of the degree of interaction, the type of facilitation, or the sequence of intervention that will lead to more functional performance (Mosey, 1981). The following are examples of postulates regarding change from a NDT standpoint:

- Crawling is enhanced by the therapist's facilitation at key points of control during play activities on the floor.
- Fine motor control is supported by stabilizing at the shoulder girdle during writing activities.

Postulates regarding change are intended to describe some type of interaction with either the human or nonhuman environment in order to facilitate function. This will lead to movement along the function-dysfunction continuum and eventual attainment of goals.

Kramer and Hinojosa (1999) provide a significant contribution to the occupational therapy literature on frames of reference for pediatric practice. This important literature enhances the profession's understanding of a particular aspect of theoretical concern in relationship to practice. However, there is still a need to provide a more holistic approach to treatment in the ever-changing demands of today's health care environments. In addition, the profession's renewed emergence of occupation-centered practice is a catalyst for promoting innovative ways of co-mingling the traditional frames of reference with broader theoretical models of practice.

Models

The term *model* has been used differently throughout a variety of professional literature. This has led to varying degrees of formality and credibility with a lack of precise meaning (Pearson, Vaughan, & FitzGerald, 2005). The interchangeable use of theory, frame of reference, and model terms within the profession also adds to the confusion when trying to explain various theoretical concepts (Braveman & Kielhofner, 2006). Mosey drew from sociological literature to describe a model in the occupational therapy profession due to its consistency with what was emerging in the profession (Mosey, 1981, 1996). Model is defined as "the typical way in which a profession perceives itself, its relationship to other professions, and its association with the society to which it is responsible" (Mosey, 1981, p. 50). Therefore, a model provides a much broader structure to view practice with children and families.

Mosey describes six key elements of a model (Table 1-2) including: philosophical assumptions, ethics, a theoretical foundation, a domain of concern, nature/principles for sequencing aspects of practice, and legitimate tools (Mosey, 1981).

Table 1-2	
SIX ELEMENTS OF A MODEL	
Philosophical Assumptions	Core beliefs about humans, their interaction with their environment, and the relationships between entities.
Ethics	Guide for moral behavior between practitioners and clients and between the profession and society.
Theoretical Foundation	Collection of theories that inform occupational therapy practice.
Domain of Concern	Aspects of importance to the profession and areas that are appropriate to provide intervention.
Nature/Principles for Sequencing Aspects of Practice	Definition and identification of problems encountered by practitioners, as well as strategies to solve them.
Legitimate Tools	The ways in which the profession is able to meet the needs of their clients.

The Person-Environment-Occupation (PEO) model (Law, Cooper, Strong, Stewart, Rigby, & Letts, 1996) is an example of a model that is effective for consideration of a more holistic viewpoint in occupational therapy. The PEO model guides an occupational therapist to consider a person's skills and abilities, the tasks and activities that are meaningful to an individual, and the environments in which engagement and participation in occupations occur. Environmental aspects that could influence occupational performance at any of these levels include cultural, institutional, physical, economic, and social factors (Law et al., 1996). Table 1-3 illustrates the elements of a model in relationship to the PEO model in order to further understand the parameters of a theoretical model in occupational therapy.

The aforementioned examples of theories, frames of reference, and models in the occupational therapy profession present a distinction that can enable practitioners to be more consistent in their language when discussing theoretical aspects. This rubric will enhance the profession's ability to more clearly delineate between a model and a frame of reference by evaluating the content of the theoretical framework. Of course there are exceptions, as noted by particular models that have evolved to incorporate aspects of a frame of reference. As the reader proceeds through the subsequent chapters, evaluation of the content will be encouraged to discuss which theoretical frameworks meet the criteria of a frame of reference or a model.

Consideration of Models for Intervention with Children and Families

Within the past decade, literature in occupational therapy regarding practice with children and families has mirrored professional advancement to more occupation-centered trends (Chapparo & Hooper, 2005; Coster, 1998). In addition, the past 20 years have

Table 1-3

EXAMPLES OF THE SIX ELEMENTS IN RELATIONSHIP TO THE
PERSON-ENVIRONMENT-OCCUPATION MODEL

Philosophical Assumptions	Occupational performance is a result of the optimal interaction of person, environment, and occupation.
Ethics	Client-centered care incorporates a respect and value for individuals and what is meaningful to them.
Theoretical Foundation	Environmental theories.
Domain of Concern	Evaluation and treatment of aspects related to the person, his or her environment, and the occupations he or she engages in.
Nature/Principles for Sequencing Aspects of Practice	Intervention for the person, environment, or occupation aspect, depending on evaluation results.
Legitimate Tools	Therapeutic use of self, meaningful activities, environmental modifications, teaching-learning process.

highlighted the recurring theme of "family-centered" practice since the legislative initiative of PL 99-457 (1986). The addition of family-centered language to primary legislation enabled occupational therapists to consider more holistic approaches. However, traditional frames of reference limit practitioners' views to considerations of the person, rather than incorporating the human and nonhuman factors, as well as the nature of occupation for individual clients. The combination of professional changes to more authentic occupational therapy and legislative initiatives that support more holistic care create an optimal time to consider models for practice in conjunction with frames of reference.

The emergence of occupational science in the 1990s has also had an impact on the profession's view of what is meaningful for individuals and their families. The study of occupations in family life is extremely valuable for understanding how individuals participate in their everyday lives. For instance, literature on mothering occupations and co-occupations inform practitioners of specific tasks and activities that are involved in the context of family operations and how women interact with their children in various situations (Esdaile & Olson, 2004). This in turn builds a bridge for understanding the unique interactions between children and their mothers in a variety of therapeutic situations.

In addition to these advancements, occupational therapists are finding themselves in unique opportunities to work in a variety of nonmedically oriented environments, such as daycares and typical preschool settings. Preventive activities in these arenas necessitate a new look at our theoretical foundations that will support innovative intervention for children, families, and alternative environments. With these various professional changes, it is important for occupational therapists working with children to expand beyond traditional frames of reference.

Models provide terms, definitions, and an organization of concepts for identifying general practice-oriented aspects that may be applied to any situation (Baum &

Christiansen, 2005). *Occupational Therapy Models for Intervention With Children and Families* is intended to create multiple ways to approach various situations in today's work environment. Chapter 2 will provide an overview of SI and NDT, the most common frames of reference in occupational intervention for children. They will be discussed in context of occupational considerations for today's practice. Subsequent chapters will provide an overview of four main models and how they can be applied to intervention with families. The text will end with a culmination chapter that describes a newer philosophical way of viewing intervention with the integration of the various models.

Learning Activity

1. Review two developmental theories, other than Piaget's Cognitive Development theory, and discuss the contribution to occupational therapy practice with children. Suggested theories include Erikson's Ego Adaptation theory, Kohlberg's Moral Development theory, and Bandura's Social Cognitive theory.

2. Review an occupational therapy frame of reference that has not been referred to in the chapter and identify the theoretical foundation, behaviors indicative of function-dysfunction, and the postulates regarding change. Kramer and Hinojosa (1999) will be a valuable resource in checking your responses. Suggested pediatric frames of reference include the Biomechanical, Psychosocial, and Coping frames of reference.

3. Explore one of the models or frames of reference in a subsequent chapter of the book. Discuss a personal rationale as to why you think it is a "model" or a "frame of reference" by integrating the parameters from Chapter 1.

References

Ayer, A. J. (2005). *Pragmatism and the meaning of the truth: The works of William James*. Cambridge, MA: Harvard University Press.

Ayres, A. J. (1989). *Sensory integration and praxis tests*. Los Angeles: Western Psychological Services.

Baum, C. M., & Christiansen, C. H. (2005). Person-environment-occupation-performance: An occupation-based framework for practice. In C. Christiansen, C. Baum, & J. Bass-Haugen (Eds.), *Occupational therapy: Performance, participation, and well-being* (p. 244). Thorofare, NJ: SLACK Incorporated.

Bobath, B. (1971). Motor development, its effect on general development and application to the treatment of cerebral palsy. *Physiotherapy, 57,* 526-532.

Braveman, B., & Kielhofner, G. (2006). Developing evidence-based occupational therapy programming. In B. Braveman (Ed.), *Leading and managing occupational therapy services* (p. 217). Philadelphia: F.A. Davis Co.

Chapparo, C. J., & Hooper, E. (2005). Self-care at school: Perceptions of 6-year-old children. *American Journal of Occupational Therapy, 59,* 67-77.

Coster, W. (1998). Occupation-centered assessment of children. *American Journal of Occupational Therapy, 52,* 337-344.

Education of the Handicapped Act Amendments of 1986 (Public Law 99-457), 20 U.S.C. 1400.

Esdaile, S. A., & Olson, J. A. (2004). *Mothering occupations: Challenge, agency, and participation*. Philadelphia: F.A. Davis Co.

Ford, D., & Urban, H. (1963). *Systems of psychotherapy*. New York: John Wiley and Sons.

Friedson, E. (1970). *Profession of medicine*. New York: Dodd, Mead and Co.

Herrick, J. (2005). *Humanism: An introduction*. Amherst, NY: Prometheus Books.

Hurff, J. (1980). A play skills inventory. A competency monitoring tool for individuals with learning deficits. *American Journal of Occupational Therapy, 34*(40), 651-656.

Kramer, P., & Hinojosa, J. (1999). *Frames of reference for pediatric occupational therapy* (2nd ed.). Philadelphia: Lippincott, Williams & Wilkins.

Kramer, P., Hinojosa, J., & Royeen, C. B. (2003). *Perspectives in human occupation: Participation in life*. Baltimore: Lippincott, Williams & Wilkins.

Law, M., Cooper, B., Strong, S., Stewart, D., Rigby, P., & Letts, L. (1996). The person-environment-occupation model: A transactive approach to occupational performance. *Canadian Journal of Occupational Therapy, 63,* 9-23.

Mosey, A. C. (1970). *Three frames of reference for mental health*. Thorofare, NJ: SLACK Incorporated.

Mosey, A. C. (1981). *Occupational therapy: Configuration of a profession*. New York: Raven Press.

Mosey, A. C. (1996). *Applied scientific inquiry in the health professions: An epistemological orientation* (2nd ed.). Bethesda, MD: American Occupational Therapy Association.

Nelson, D. L., & Jepson-Thomas, J. (2003). Occupational form, occupational performance, and a conceptual framework for therapeutic occupation. In P. Kramer, J., Hinojosa, & C. B. Royeen (Eds.), *Perspectives in human occupation: Participation in life*. Baltimore: Lippincott, Williams & Wilkins.

Pearson, A., Vaughan, B., & FitzGerald, M. (2005). *Nursing models for practice* (3rd ed.). New York: Butterworth-Heinemann.

Peloquin, S. (2000). The philosophy of occupational therapy. In A. Punwar & S. Peloquin (Eds.), *Occupational therapy: Principles and practice* (3rd ed., pp. 7-20). Baltimore: Lippincott, Williams & Wilkins.

Piaget, J. (1950). *The psychology of intelligence*. London: Routledge & Kegan Paul.

Reilly, M. (1966). The challenge of the future to an occupational therapist. *American Journal of Occupational Therapy, 20,* 221-225.

Reilly, M. (1969). The education process. *American Journal of Occupational Therapy, 23,* 299-307.

Schoen, S. A., & Anderson, J. (1999). NeuroDevelopmental treatment and frame of reference. In P. Kramer & J. Hinojosa (Eds.), *Frames of reference for pediatric occupational therapy* (2nd ed., pp. 83-118). Baltimore: Lippincott, Williams & Wilkins.

Thomas, R. M. (1999). *Human development theories: Windows on culture*. Thousand Oaks, CA: Sage Publications Inc.

Walker, L. O., & Avant, K. C. (1995). *Strategies for theory construction in nursing* (3rd ed.). Englewood Cliffs, NJ: Prentice Hall.

2

SENSORY INTEGRATION AND NEURODEVELOPMENTAL TREATMENT AS FRAMES OF REFERENCE IN THE CONTEXT OF OCCUPATIONAL SCIENCE

Erna Imperatore Blanche, PhD, OTR/L, FAOTA
Dominique Blanche Kiefer, OTD, OTR/L

Learning Objectives

At the end of this chapter, the reader will be able to:
- Describe occupational science as a context for occupational therapy interventions/frames of reference.
- Identify basic concepts of Sensory Integration (SI) as a frame of reference and its relationship to occupational science.
- Identify basic concepts of Neurodevelopmental Treatment (NDT) and its relationship to occupational science.
- Apply NDT and SI concepts of intervention within the context of occupational science.
- Relate occupational science research to occupational therapy with children and their families.

Introduction

The issues presented by children with disabilities and their families are complex and require understanding of multiple levels of performance. In order to address these complexities, the clinician needs to consider the child's functional limitations while focusing on how these limitations impact occupational performance and participation in the family's activities. Successful intervention of these multiple layers of function requires the use of multiple frames of reference, theories, and models. This chapter describes the two most often-utilized pediatric frames of reference, Sensory Integration (SI) and

Neurodevelopmental Treatment (NDT), and their use as intervention approaches within an occupational science perspective and occupational science-based practice. NDT and SI as frames of reference address the child's functional limitations, while research from occupational science can guide the intervention toward successful engagement in daily occupations and participation in the community. Understanding frames of reference is critical for comparisons to theoretical models in subsequent chapters, as well as for gaining an appreciation of the possibilities of combining and integrating the use of frames and models.

Defining and Comparing Concepts

SENSORY INTEGRATION AND NEURODEVELOPMENTAL TREATMENT

As mentioned in Chapter 1, NDT and SI are two of the most widely utilized frames of reference in pediatrics. However, before utilizing these approaches, it is important to consider that these two frames of reference are distinctly different in at least three ways: their theoretical foundations, the founding discipline, and the evolution of the approach.

From a theoretical point of view, Ayres initially intended for her research in SI to be a theory providing explanations for human behavior and not necessarily a frame of reference for intervention (Ayres, 1979). Furthermore, Ayres developed a standardized assessment tool to identify and describe how sensory processing played a role in the normal development of the child and how inefficient processing resulted in decreased participation in daily occupations (Ayres, 1972b, 1989). Only after Ayres described the unusual patterns of sensory processing was she able to develop a frame of reference for intervention that was firmly rooted in the occupation of play (Ayres, 1972b). On the other hand, NDT from its inception was developed as a frame of reference for intervention for a known disorder, cerebral palsy. Berta and Karel Bobath intended this approach as an alternative to the treatment strategies utilized with children with cerebral palsy at the time. They focused on understanding the postural and movement impairments of children with cerebral palsy, thus the focal point of intervention was on those aspects of performance (Bly, 1983; Bobath & Bobath, 1975).

Examining the founding discipline of each of these frames of reference also reveals differences between them. SI was developed within the profession of occupational therapy with a focus centered on occupation. A physical therapist and a physician within the context of those professions developed NDT. At first, NDT did not incorporate functional performance or occupation; therefore, when occupational therapists adopted this frame of reference instead of moving NDT strategies toward occupation, they moved toward analysis of movement components such as reflexes, postural control, and muscle tone (Blanche & Hallway, 1998; Fiorentino, 1966). Soon after, Finnie (1975) offered a fresh approach to NDT intervention by including parent training in handling the children during their daily routines at home. It was during the later years that the occupational therapists adopting NDT learned to infuse functional performance and occupation into its context.

Lastly, the evolution of both SI and NDT from their inceptions offered different perspectives of the child's occupational performance. SI provides an explanation of sensory processes affecting motor performance, learning, and behavior, while NDT offers an explanation of the components of motor performance that may hinder the child's participation in society. Their evolution is also markedly different. SI can be considered a theory and a frame of reference. As a theory, it offers explanations of the relationship between sensory processing and observable behaviors. As mentioned in Chapter 1, the relationships offered by theories provide predictions of behavior under certain circum-stances (Mosey, 1981). This is applicable to SI theory, which predicts behaviors that relate to sensory processing.

SI can also be viewed as a frame of reference because it offers a unique intervention in which therapists focus on the sensory experience and the performance that needs to be challenged within a context of play and social interaction. SI treatment includes all four specific characteristics outlined in Chapter 1, including a theoretical base, function-dys-function continuum, description of behaviors indicative of function and dysfunction, and postulates regarding change. In addition, this approach honors the importance of intrin-sic motivation as well as the relationship with the therapist, both of which are firmly rooted in the philosophical beliefs of the founders of occupational therapy.

As with other frames of reference used in pediatric practices, its effectiveness is still moderately supported with research (Ayres, 1972a; Humpries, Snider, & McDougall, 1993). However, the presence of SI deficits in children with a variety of disorders is more firmly supported with empirical evidence (Ayres, 1989; Baranek, Foster, & Berkson, 1997; Cermak & Daunhauer, 1997; Dunn, Myles, & Orr, 2002; Miller, Reisman, McIntosh, & Simon, 2001; Mulligan, 1996; Parham, 1998).

As mentioned in Chapter 1, NDT is considered a frame of reference for intervention. It certainly provides the aforementioned four primary aspects that characterize a frame of reference. When first developed, NDT offered an innovative analysis of the movement disorders in children with cerebral palsy and an intervention approach rooted in this analysis. Although the analysis is recognized as a tool in the evaluation process, the effec-tiveness of the intervention approach has moderate support in research (Fetters & Kluzik, 1996; Jonsdottir, Fetters, & Kluzik, 1997; Law, Cadman, Rosenbaum, Walter, Russell, & DeMatteo, 1991).

Occupational Science

Occupational science is neither a theory, frame of reference, nor a model. It is a basic and applied science that offers theoretical explanations and research on various aspects of occupation (Carlson & Dunlea, 1995; Clark et al., 1991; Yerxa et al., 1989; Zemke & Clark, 1996). Findings from occupational science research can provide a framework illustrating the complexity of occupation and the opportunity for the development of theories, frames of reference, and models to emanate from it. Initially, Clark and Larson (1993) presented a hierarchical model of the human that organized knowledge areas in occupational sci-ence and occupational therapy. Although it was not intended as a model for intervention, this model could help practitioners conceptualize the patient's areas of limitations and its impact to occupational performance. Later, Clark (1993; Clark, Ennevor, & Richardson, 1996) and Jackson and colleagues (1998) directly applied occupational science research findings to clinical practice, creating what is known as Lifestyle Redesign™ and thus expanding the borders of occupational therapy. This application of occupational sci-ence research to occupational therapy practice became what is informally referred to as "occupational science-based practice" or practice that is based on occupational science research. Lifestyle Redesign with diverse populations and direct cultural interventions (Frank et al., 2001; Mandel, Jackson, Zemke, Nelson, & Clark, 1999) are two clinical pro-grams that exemplify occupational science-based practice.

Pierce, another occupational scientist, offers a slightly different application of occupa-tional science to clinical practice. In what can be considered a frame of reference, Pierce identifies occupation as a "modality for intervention" (2003, p. 8) and describes a process for becoming effective designers of occupation-based interventions. This approach to intervention is firmly rooted in occupational science and offers clinicians a roadmap to the creation of occupation-based intervention. These examples provide a glimpse to the different ways that occupational science can inform clinical practice.

A distinction must be made between occupational science-based practice and occupation-based practice. In this text, we will refer to occupational science-based practice as models, frames of reference, or intervention programs that are based on occupational science research. It differs from occupation-based practice in that it is centered on the literature emanating from occupational science. Occupation-based practice is founded on the philosophical belief that occupation is essential for the well-being of the individual. Treatment using an occupation-based practice approach centers on occupation but is not necessarily based on basic or applied occupational science research. However, in both instances, models and frames of reference developed within or outside the profession can be incorporated in the intervention process.

When focusing on the occupation of the child and the family, occupational science offers pertinent research that can be used concurrently with pediatric approaches such as NDT and SI in clinical practice. In this chapter, two conceptual maps illustrating the use of SI and NDT as frames of reference for intervention within the context of occupation-based practice and occupational science research are presented. These models allow for the inclusion of occupational science research and frames of reference for intervention in order to provide a richer perspective of the child's difficulties in the context of the family. In the same manner, Gray (1998) describes occupation-based practice as using occupation as the means and the outcome of intervention. NDT and SI contribute to the development of occupational performance as component-focused tools of intervention in the context of play and other functional occupations.

An Occupational Science Conceptual Map

The first conceptual map illustrating the relationship between occupational science, SI, and NDT is presented in Figure 2-1. It is based on systems theory, motor control theories, concepts from occupational science, and the International Classification of Functioning, Disability, and Health (World Health Organization, 2001). This conceptual map provides a general viewpoint for organizing the multiple elements that contribute to the performance of occupation. Although this conceptual map has similarities with the Person-Environment-Occupation (PEO) model, it also has a clear and distinct difference. The conceptual map presented in Figure 2-1 depicts occupation as the outcome of the interaction between the person, the environment, and the task requirements, while the PEO model illustrates occupation as a separate aspect from the person and the environment.

Furthermore, in occupational science, *form* refers to the observable aspect of an occupation; *function* refers to the service of occupation toward development, adaptation, and health; and *meaning* refers to the subjective experience linked to the significance of the occupation in the person's life (Clark, Wood, & Larson, 1998; Larson, Wood, & Clark, 2003). This conceptual map depicts the relationship between the person, the task requirements, and the environment as part of the form of the occupation. People derive the function of the occupation from their trajectory through time (short- and long-term), and they derive meaning from their experience of the occupation. For example, the occupation of "playing soccer" is the product of the person, environment (physical, cultural, social), and task requirements (sensory, neuromotor, etc.). But "playing soccer" is recognized by the form of the occupation. The function may likely change over the course of a person's lifetime, from playing competitively as a child to playing recreationally for health reasons as the person ages. Likewise, the meaning of "playing soccer" lies within the individual and may change over time.

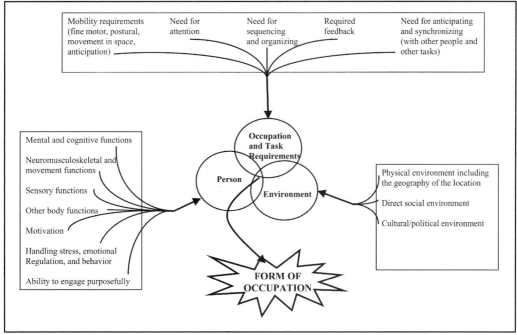

Figure 2-1. Conceptual map. (Adapted from Blanche, E. I., & Kiefer, D. B. [2006]. Unpublished document.)

Learning Activity A

1. Pick from the following experiences and describe form, function, and meaning from your own personal perspective:
   - Family dining at their favorite restaurant after a school play
   - Neighborhood soccer play during middle childhood
   - First driving experience
   - Siblings playing cards
2. Describe two experiences related to intervention with clients and discuss possible form, function, and meaning aspects from the following examples:
   - Kendall, a 3-year-old girl with spastic cerebral palsy, finger feeding at preschool
   - Jackson, a 7-year-old boy, repeatedly runs into peers during an outdoor physical education class
3. Describe the possible NDT and SI aspects of consideration in the two examples given in #2.
   - Describe the possible physical, social, and cultural environmental factors that will influence participation in occupations for the examples in #2 (or for your own examples).

When examining the conceptual map presented in Figure 2-1, three key elements contribute to the performance of occupation. The first is the person's attributes, such as sensory processing functions, neuromusculoskeletal and movement functions, mental and cognitive functions, other body functions, motivation, capacity to handle stress, emotional regulation, and the ability to engage purposefully. Clinicians have traditionally utilized SI and NDT to address performance from this perspective. Therapists using an SI frame of reference evaluate how each of these components are affected by the sensory input in the environment and how a child interprets and regulates the information. The evaluation and treatment for children with SI dysfunctions are often focused on their sensory functions, their ability to move, motivation, capacity to handle stress, and emotional regulation emanating from sensory input in the environment as well as their ability to engage in purposeful tasks. NDT focuses on the neuromusculoskeletal and movement functions affecting participation as well as the environmental limitations to functional performance.

The second key element contributing to the performance of occupation are the task requirements, including mobility requirements (fine motor, gross motor, postural control, stability, and mobility in space), the need for focused attention, the need for sequencing and organizing (continuous vs. discrete), the need for feedback (open and closed-looped tasks), and the need for anticipating and synchronizing actions with other people and with other tasks. When utilizing SI or NDT as a frame of reference, clinicians often need to take into account the requirements of the task presented to the child. For example, running on the beach is a task that requires continuous movement but little anticipation, while playing ball with friends requires constant feedback and anticipation as well as focused attention and synchronizing actions with others. Children with sensory processing problems may not have any difficulties running, but often have difficulty playing ball with friends.

Lastly, the environment characteristics also contribute to the form of the occupation. This includes the physical environment (e.g., the geography of the neighborhood, the accessibility to transportation, competing multiple events, technology available), the social context (e.g., attitudes of others, social support, social interaction), and the cultural and political aspects of the environment (e.g., cultural practices, services available, policies affecting reimbursement). The family is one of the most important environmental influences in the lives of children, because the information to which they are exposed and the opportunities they will have will largely depend on their families.

RELATIONSHIP TO OCCUPATIONAL SCIENCE RESEARCH

With the interaction of these three key elements, performance in occupation arises. The occupational science research illustrates that participation and engagement in occupation is further complicated when considering enfolded occupations and the importance of synchronizing actions when engaging in co-occupations such as breastfeeding (Dunlea, 1996; Larson & Zemke, 2003). Research in occupational science can help occupational therapists understand this issue when addressing children with disabilities and their families. For example, Primeau (1998) describes how parents of children without disabilities often enfold occupations such as incorporating play into their daily routines. During these occupations, the purpose of enfolding play may be for their children to learn new tasks. Primeau (1998) refers to the teaching of tasks within a daily routine as scaffolding. On the other hand, research with parents of children with disabilities reveals that parents may have difficulty performing daily simultaneous occupations that other parents do automatically, and rather than enfold occupations, they tend to unfold or break the occupations into smaller chunks in order to complete them (Segal, 2000). Research in occupational science has also shown that parents of children with disabilities may choose to allow children to perform occupations that therapists ask to discontinue because those occupations may "nourish" their children's sensory needs (Blanche, 2001).

GENERAL IMPLICATIONS FOR PRACTICE

Occupational therapists utilizing SI and NDT as frames of reference often include aspects of parent instruction. In this situation, incorporating the previously mentioned research may provide therapists with guidelines on how parents of children with disabilities can actually include their recommendations. For example, rather than add tasks to the parents' already overloaded day, therapists may teach the parents to unfold or break the daily occupations into smaller chunks that can be completed when the children are in bed. Therapists can also encourage parents to understand their children's sensory needs and use these sensory needs when entering with them into play. This may lead to a greater enjoyment of the family life rather than having parents follow a rigorous intervention routine.

In addition to enfolding and unfolding occupations, synchronizing actions is important in occupations such as feeding an infant, catching a ball, and arriving on time to have lunch with a friend. In family life, their style of interacting, occupational engagement, and synchronizing simultaneous and sequential family occupations becomes pivotal when assessing and intervening with children with disabilities. For example, a child with SI disorders in a large family may need to learn to adapt to their rapid speed in order to fully participate in the family's routine. In this case, the therapist may utilize SI techniques that help the child deal with competing sensory events as well as teach the child compensatory patterns to organize his or her routine so he or she can follow the family's schedule. On the other hand, a family's rapid routine may need to accommodate the needs of a child with cerebral palsy. The therapist may teach the parents some basic NDT handling techniques to make the daily occupations of feeding and dressing easier and more enjoyable. Therefore, the person, environment, and task requirements influence not only the participation and performance in occupation, but also the ability to synchronize with other people and engage in co-occupations.

This conceptual map also provides an outline for intervention using SI and NDT frames of reference. For example, an SI dysfunction would be identified as part of the person, however, its expression would depend on the task and the environment in which the person is participating. As seen in the examples provided previously, a therapist can choose to intervene by changing the child's sensory processing or reaction to events or by providing environmental modifications (changing the task requirements or the environment the child is in). If these therapists were using NDT as the primary frame of reference, then the treatment approach would traditionally be centered at the level of the person; however the analysis utilized in NDT would allow the therapist to identify tasks that would be difficult for the child to perform and how to modify the home and school environment to maximize performance and participation in occupation.

Learning Activity B

1. Review two other occupational science research articles related to children and families.
2. Discuss how the information from these articles can inform practice for children with developmental issues and their families.

Practice Utilizing Occupational Science Research, Models of Practice, and Frames of Reference for Intervention

Figure 2-2 outlines the second conceptual map presented in this chapter. However, this map is directed at organizing the intervention. It depicts the process of understanding a child's difficulties using a method for gathering information and planning intervention from a holistic point of view that takes into consideration the child in the context of the family and their participation in everyday occupations. In this figure, NDT and SI are included in the evaluation and the intervention phases, while the process is guided by an understanding of the need to ultimately focus on the child's and the family's occupations and their participation in the community. For that, an understanding of models of practice, as well as occupational science concepts and research findings, will guide the process. NDT and SI, as well as the evidence supporting these frames of reference, will focus on specific aspects contributing to the performance of occupations.

EVALUATION AND ANALYSIS

The reason for referral to occupational therapy often includes limited participation in occupations. Analysis of these occupations may shed light on the evaluation tools that can be utilized. Standardized and nonstandardized evaluation tools used within NDT and SI often focus on body functions that are difficult for the child; however, evaluation tools of the child's well-being could be included in the evaluation process as well. Analysis of performance, based on SI and NDT, can also be utilized to examine the child's participation in chosen tasks and in specific environments. The analysis of movement that is part of NDT can be used to understand how the task and the environment need adjustment for the child to function optimally. For example, the child may need a higher desk or an angled seat in order to maintain adequate body alignment during writing skills. In addition, SI as a theory can be used in the evaluation phase to understand the children's sensory processing difficulties, as well as the impact of the environmental stimuli on their performance.

During the evaluation phase, interviews and questionnaires with the parents can shed light on the child's birth history and sensory history, as well as on the family's narrative of their child's difficulties and their importance in the context of their family life. The clinician can also gather understanding of the child's and the parent's preferred occupations and play style (Blanche, 2001; Knox, 1996). Incorporating an understanding of the preferred occupations and play styles will allow the therapist to include them successfully in the intervention process with the child, as well as with the family's recreation choices.

TREATMENT PLANNING

Once the evaluation is complete, the therapist and the family can choose the best possible plan of action based on the present and future expectations. The plan of action needs to include the evidence supporting the intervention. Evidence may emanate from occupational science, the child's difficulties that need to be addressed, or from the child's limitations. Throughout this process, SI and NDT play a role in the analysis and the intervention of the child's functional limitations. Understanding SI as a theory can also influence the choice of occupations that are prescribed. For example, a child who is fidgety and restless may present a reduced response to proprioceptive input and thus may benefit from engaging in occupations that provide this input such as jumping on a trampoline and rock climbing. These occupations could provide the child with the input he or she

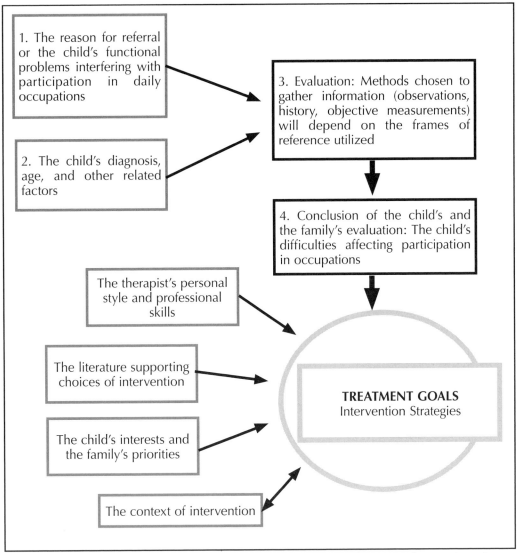

Figure 2-2. Information that needs to be taken into consideration during clinical reasoning. Two-sided arrows indicate the links between the information that is gathered. One-sided arrows depict vital information that leads to the formation of the working hypothesis. For example, the child's functional problems interfering with participation in daily occupations are labeled (1), and the child's diagnosis, age, and related factors are labeled (2). These two sources of information are necessary in order to decide the method utilized to gather information, which is numbered (3). (Adapted from Blanche, E. I. [2003]. *Gathering information to design successful intervention programs.* Unpublished manuscript.)

needs, while remaining engaged in meaningful choices of play and recreation. Research on play can also be used to guide the context and organization of the intervention. For example, allowing the child to choose and incorporating play elements into the session will make the therapeutic occupations more meaningful and enjoyable for the child.

Lastly, research in clinical reasoning and occupational science also illustrates the importance of incorporating the therapist's self-reflection on attitudes and expectations as part of the social environment. The therapist's narrative influences the therapeutic process and requires awareness as the child's story is built by the child, family, and therapist (Burke, 2001; Clark, 1993; Lawlor, 2003).

Lifestyle Redesign

This chapter has provided some basic ideas of how to incorporate occupational science research and SI and NDT as frames of reference into practice. In this section, occupational science-based practice that has been modified for children with SI disorders and their families will be presented. Occupational science-based practice endorses the use of occupational science research in the development of innovative practice.

The most popular approach based on occupational science research is Lifestyle Redesign. This approach was initially developed for the healthy aging population but has been applied to the treatment of obesity and other health-related problems. Lifestyle Redesign can also be used to address the lifestyle issues of children with SI dysfunction. In this case, the program would include parents and families in a group situation and would evaluate and discuss the match between the parent's and the child's sensory style. The result is an intervention program in which the families, in conjunction with the professionals, create strategies that address the child's sensory needs in the home and the community and thus decrease behavioral issues. Table 2-1 presents one of the programs based on this concept.

Conclusion

Addressing the complex issues presented by children with disabilities and their families requires inclusion of intervention strategies at multiple levels of performance. Successful occupational therapy practice focuses not only on the child's limitations but also on the family's values, interests, and lifestyle choices. Hence, the intervention requires addressing the children's limitations while maximizing their occupational performance within the family and the community. This chapter describes the use of two pediatric frames of reference (SI and NDT) within the context of occupation and occupational science research findings. SI and NDT as frames of reference address the child's functional limitations, and occupational science research can provide a guide for intervention. The opportunity to provide a more effective and holistic intervention is embedded in the use of multiple strategies.

The following cases illustrate the concepts presented in this chapter. They highlight the use of SI and NDT in addressing functional limitations in a play- and occupation-rich environment. The development of these skills translated into increased participation in family and community life. By embedding SI and NDT into therapeutic occupations of play, the therapist helps the child engage independently in these and other play occupations at home and in the community.

Table 2-1
But Why? Family Link Program

Program Description

This program is geared toward families with children with sensory processing difficulties affecting movement and behavior. The program consists of four sessions during which the parents are guided through the identification of their own sensory needs and their children's sensory processing difficulties, as well as possible strategies that can be used to address difficult behaviors. The program utilizes lectures, exercises, videotaped sessions, group discussions, and observations of parent-child interactions.

Purpose and Goals

To train parents to identify behaviors that relate to sensory processing and to address their children's sensory needs by using simple modifications of the physical and social environment.

Methods

Four weekly meetings of small groups of parents (three to six parents per group). Methods utilized to present information include handouts, discussions, practical exercises, video-taped observations of parent-child interactions during play, and therapeutic feedback during unstructured play situations.

Description of Each Session

Session 1

This session focuses on typical development of sensory processing and its effect on movement and behavior. The theory of SI is used as a frame of reference to discuss this topic. Methods of education include discussions, practical exercises, observations, discussion of parent responses in sensory surveys, and handouts. Parents are asked to identify problem behaviors at home, determine possible strategies to address these behaviors, and bring them up for discussion during Week 2.

> *Purpose*
> - To discuss the sensory self by helping the parents recognize their own sensory needs and avoidances.
> - To understand the influence of sensory processing on functional and not-so-functional skills.
> - To identify signs of sensory stressors and their impact on well-being and participation in everyday life.

Session 2

This session focuses on parents' reports of behaviors observed at home and in the community and on strategies to address them. The group analyzes the parents' videos of their children and provides ideas about strategies for intervention. The group also discusses sensory stressors, sensory strategies, and environment modifications to address children's needs.

Case Study #1: Sebastian

When Nora Romano first called requesting intervention for her 1-year-old son, Sebastian, she sounded frustrated. She described him as a lively child, but she had suspected from the beginning that something was wrong. He was born at 9 months gestation and, with the exception of a car accident during her pregnancy, her pregnancy was uneventful. Sebastian was described as a "good baby" who did not move much. As the fourth child in this family, Nora welcomed his nondemanding nature; however, when he was 7 months old, she noticed that he was moving his left side less than the right. His random arm and leg movements appeared asymmetrical and he only grasped a cookie with his right hand. It had taken 2 months for the pediatrician to refer the child to physical therapy and from there to occupational therapy.

The Romano family was a lively group. The three older children (ages 9, 7, and 5) were active in extracurricular activities and family activities. Nora loved hiking and camping from when she was a teen and had maintained this activity throughout the birth of all four children. As a family, they enjoyed hiking and often camped as part of their family vacations.

The initial evaluation revealed that Sebastian had neuromotor difficulties that needed to be addressed with NDT. In this case, SI became a secondary frame of reference. The therapist explained that Sebastian would need intervention in order to be able to freely move in space and participate in activities such as dressing himself and climbing the structures in the park. The therapist suggested weekly sessions to address the upper extremity difficulties as well as some incipient motor planning difficulties.

The weekly treatment sessions focused on helping Sebastian acquire the ability to incorporate the left hand in bimanual activities. The therapist used NDT to address postural control, dynamic weight bearing on the upper extremities, bilateral reach, and hand manipulation skills while Sebastian bounced on the ball, popped bubbles, played with blocks, or banged a musical toy. In addition, she provided home environment and community modifications so Sebastian could sit with the family at the table and participate in the weekly hiking trips.

As Sebastian progressed and his motor skills improved, his sensory processing and motor planning limitations became more apparent. The therapist then switched to an SI frame of reference. Sebastian now walked independently in the clinic and home environment, so the therapist used gross motor play to engage him in activities that challenged his postural control and motor planning skills. At home, he could now participate actively in the hiking trips as he walked on the path.

Case Study #2: Marcelo

Joaquin Sanchez found out about SI from a parenting course he attended when his child, Marcelo, was 6 years old. At that time, Joaquin figured out that his child's performance in school could be improved. Joaquin described Marcelo as having difficulty attending, getting dressed, learning to write, and participating in other classroom and playground activities. He was constantly in motion, running, climbing, and chasing other children. The school had denied services because Marcelo's performance was not significantly below the other kindergarteners in his class. Marcelo's teacher believed that these difficulties were "behavioral" and asked the parents to be firmer with the boy. Although

Joaquin had recently emigrated from Mexico and could barely speak English, he knew by the teacher's tone of voice that she believed he was not a good father because his child was "out of control." Joaquin's rationale was that if they were not good parents, then their other child would also be "out of control" and that was not the case. Joaquin worked as a janitor in a bank. His wife, Ofelia, worked part time as a housekeeper and seamstress. She did not drive.

After his meeting with the teacher, Joaquin decided he needed to find out more about his child's behavior so he attended the "But Why? Family Link Program," which was a free class for parents about incorporating SI principles in the home setting. He then realized that maybe some of his son's behaviors were sensory based and requested an independent occupational therapy evaluation.

Mariana, the occupational therapist assigned to Marcelo, had learned Spanish and lived in Guatemala when she was in high school. Mariana had been trained as a behaviorist before she became proficient in SI. Mariana observed Marcelo during writing, circle time, and while participating on the playground. She noticed that Marcelo sat on the back of his heels and jumped up and down at least 60% of the time when sitting in circle time. He sometimes turned around and disrupted the other children. During handwriting, Marcelo needed to stand and walk around continuously, something that the parents reported he did also during meal times at home. In the playground, Marcelo spent his time chasing children, swinging, and twirling. A questionnaire focusing on home and school occupations provided to the parents and further clinical evaluation revealed hyporesponsiveness to vestibular and proprioceptive input. Mariana suggested weekly consultation with the teacher and some school modifications. Based on the evidence available, she decided to order a weighted vest and an inflatable ball for Marcelo to sit on during class.

Mariana was aware that Marcelo also needed individual services, however, the funding system only offered consultation at this time. Mariana then provided Marcelo's parents with a daily sensory diet to help incorporate sensory input into daily occupations and invited them to participate in the Family Link program.

With the help of the consultations and attending the Family Link program, the parents learned to incorporate a sensory diet into the family routine. Marcelo lived in a poor neighborhood that had a small park three blocks away. Mariana and Marcelo's mother developed a routine for the family to go to the park at least 3 days a week. At home, he sat on an inflatable ball when doing his homework and when watching TV. Marcelo also participated in a tutoring program after school.

References

Ayres, A. J. (1972a). Improving academic scores through sensory integration. *Journal of Learning Disabilities, 5,* 336-343.

Ayres, A. J. (1972b). *Sensory integration and learning disorders.* Los Angeles: Western Psychological Services.

Ayres, A. J. (1979). *Sensory integration and the child.* Los Angeles: Western Psychological Services.

Ayres, A. J. (1989). *Sensory integration and praxis test—SIPT manual.* Los Angeles: Western Psychological Services.

Baranek, G. T., Foster, L. G., & Berkson, G. (1997). Tactile defensiveness and stereotyped behaviors. *American Journal of Occupational Therapy, 51,* 91-95.

Blanche, E. I. (2001). Transformative occupations and long-range adaptive responses. In S. Smith-Roley, E. Blanche, & R. Schaaf (Eds.), *Sensory integration with diverse populations* (pp. 421-432). San Antonio, TX: Therapy Skill Builders.

Blanche, E. I., & Hallway, M. (1998). Historical perspective: Neurodevelopmental treatment in occupational therapy. *Developmental Disabilities Special Interest Section Quarterly, 21*(3), 1-3.

Bly, L. (1983). *The components of normal movement during the first year of life and abnormal motor development* (monograph). Chicago: NDTA.

Bobath, K., & Bobath, B. (1975). *Motor development in the different types of cerebral palsy.* London: William Heineman Medical Books, Ltd.

Burke, J. (2001). Clinical reasoning and the use of narrative in sensory integration assessment and intervention. In S. Smith-Roley, E. Blanche, & R. Schaaf (Eds.), *Sensory integration with diverse populations* (pp. 203-212). San Antonio, TX: Therapy Skill Builders.

Carlson, M., & Dunlea, A. (1995). Further thoughts on the pitfalls of partition: A response to Mosey. *American Journal of Occupational Therapy, 49,* 73-81.

Cermak, S. A., & Daunhauer, L. A. (1997). Sensory processing in the postinstitutionalized child. *American Journal of Occupational Therapy, 51,* 500-506.

Clark, F. (1993). Occupation embedded in a real life: Interweaving occupational science and occupational therapy. *American Journal of Occupational Therapy, 47,* 1067-1078.

Clark, F., Ennevor, B. L., & Richardson, P. L. (1996). A grounded theory of techniques for occupational storytelling and occupational storymaking. In R. Zemke & F. Clark (Eds.), *Occupational science: The evolving discipline* (pp. 373-392). Philadelphia: F.A. Davis Co.

Clark, F., & Larson, E. (1993). Developing an academic discipline: The science of occupation. In H. Hopkins & H. Smith (Eds.), *Willard and Spackman's occupational therapy* (8th ed., pp. 44-55). Philadelphia: J.B. Lippincott Co.

Clark, F., Parham, D., Carlson, M., Frank, G., Jackson, J., Pierce, D., Wolfe, R., & Zemke, R. (1991). Occupational science: Academic innovation in the service of occupational therapy's future. *American Journal of Occupational Therapy, 45,* 300-310.

Clark, F., Wood, W., & Larson, E. (1998). Occupational science: Occupational therapy's legacy for the 21st century. In M. E. Neistadt & E. B. Crepeau (Eds.), *Willard and Spackman's occupational therapy* (9th ed., pp. 13-21). Philadelphia: J.B. Lippincott Co.

Dunlea, A. (1996). An opportunity for co-occupation: The experience of mother and their infants who are blind. In R. Zemke & F. Clark (Eds.), *Occupational science: The evolving discipline.* Philadelphia: F.A. Davis Co.

Dunn, W., Myles, B. S., & Orr, S. (2002). Sensory processing issues associated with Asperger syndrome: A preliminary investigation. *American Journal of Occupational Therapy, 56,* 97-102.

Fetters, L., & Kluzik, J. (1996). The effects of neurodevelopmental treatment versus practice on the reaching of children with spastic cerebral palsy. *Physical Therapy, 76,* 346-358.

Finnie, N. (1975). *Handling the young cerebral palsied child at home.* New York: E.P. Dutton and Co., Inc.

Fiorentino, M. R. (1966). The changing dimension of occupational therapy. *American Journal of Occupational Therapy, 20*(5), 251-252.

Frank, G., Fishman, M., Crowley, C., Blair, B., Murphy, S. T., Montoya, J. A., Hickey, M. P., Brancaccio, M. V., & Bensimon, E. M. (2001). The new stories/new cultures after-school enrichment program: A direct cultural intervention. *American Journal of Occupational Therapy, 55,* 501-508.

Gray, J. M. (1998). Putting occupation into practice: Occupation as ends, occupation as means. *American Journal of Occupational Therapy, 52,* 354-364.

Humpries, T., Snider, L., & McDougall, B. (1993). Clinical evaluation of the effectiveness of sensory integrative and perceptual motor therapy in improving sensory integrative function in children with learning disabilities. *Occupational Therapy Journal of Research, 13*(3), 163-182.

Jackson, J., Carlson, M., Mandel, D., Zemke, R., & Clark, F. (1998). Occupation in lifestyle redesign: The well elderly study occupational therapy program. *American Journal of Occupational Therapy, 52,* 326-336.

Jonsdottir, J., Fetters, L., & Kluzik, J. (1997). Effects of physical therapy on postural control in children with cerebral palsy. *Pediatric Physical Therapy, 9,* 69-75.

Knox, S. H. (1996). Play and playfulness in preschool children. In R. Zemke & F. Clark (Eds.), *Occupational science: The evolving discipline* (pp. 81-88). Philadelphia: F.A. Davis Co.

Larson, E., Wood, W., & Clark, F. (2003). Occupational science: Building the science and practice of occupation through an academic discipline. In E. Crepeau, E. Cohn, & B. Schell (Eds.), *Willard and Spackman's occupational therapy* (10th ed.). Philadelphia: Lippincott, Williams & Wilkins.

Larson, E., & Zemke, R. (2003). Shaping the temporal patterns of our lives: The social coordination of occupation. *Journal of Occupational Science, 10*(2), 80-89.

Law, M., Cadman, D., Rosenbaum, P., Walter, S., Russell, D., & DeMatteo, C. (1991). Neurodevelopmental therapy and upper-extremity inhibitive casting for children with cerebral palsy. *Developmental Medicine and Child Neurology, 33,* 379-387.

Lawlor, M. (2003). The significance of being occupied: The social construction of childhood occupations. *American Journal of Occupational Therapy, 57*(4), 424-434.

Mandel, D. R., Jackson, J. M., Zemke, R., Nelson, L., & Clark, F. A. (1999). *Lifestyle Redesign: Implementing the well elderly program*. Bethesda, MD: American Occupational Therapy Association.

Miller, L. J., Reisman, J., McIntosh, D. N., & Simon, J. (2001). An ecological model of sensory modulation: Performance of children with fragile X syndrome, autistic disorder, attention-deficit/hyperactivity disorder, and sensory modulation dysfunction. In S. Smith-Roley, E. Blanche, & R. Schaaf (Eds.), *Understanding the nature of sensory integration with diverse populations* (pp. 57-85). San Antonio, TX: Therapy Skill Builders.

Mosey, A. C. (1981). *Occupational therapy: Configuration of a profession.* New York: Raven Press.

Mulligan, S. (1996). An analysis of score patterns of children with attention disorders on the sensory integration and praxis tests. *American Journal of Occupational Therapy, 50*(8), 647–654.

Parham, L. D. (1998). The relationship of sensory integrative development to achievement in elementary students: Four-year longitudinal patterns. *Occupational Therapy Journal of Research, 18*(3), 105-127.

Pierce, D. (2003). *Occupation by design–Building therapeutic power.* Philadelphia: F.A. Davis Co.

Primeau, L. (1998). Orchestration of work and play within families. *American Journal of Occupational Therapy, 52*(3), 188-195.

Segal, R. (2000). Adaptive strategies of mothers with children with attention deficit hyperactivity disorder: Enfolding and unfolding occupations. *American Journal of Occupational Therapy, 54*(3), 300-306.

World Health Organization. (2001). *International classification of functioning, disability, and health.* Geneva, Switzerland: Author.

Yerxa, E. J., Clark, F., Frank, G., Jackson, J., Parham, D., Pierce, D., Stein, C., & Zemke, R. (1989). An introduction to occupational science: A foundation for occupational therapy in the 21st century. *Occupational Therapy in Health Care, 6,* 1-17.

Zemke, R., & Clark, F. (1996). Preface. In R. Zemke & F. Clark (Eds.), *Occupational science: The evolving discipline* (pp. vii-xviii). Philadelphia: F.A. Davis Co.

PERSON-ENVIRONMENT-OCCUPATION MODEL

Mary Law, PhD, OT(C)
Sandra Barker Dunbar, DPA, OTR/L

Learning Objectives

At the end of this chapter, the reader will be able to:
- Identify the theoretical foundations of the Person-Environment-Occupation (PEO) model.
- Analyze the person, environment, and/or occupation factors that influence performance of occupations of children and youth.
- Select assessment tools that identify occupational performance issues within the context of the PEO model.
- Create intervention plans that address the person, environment, and/or occupation realms within the PEO model.
- Apply a family-centered approach to occupational therapy intervention.

— SECTION I —

Overview of the Person-Environment-Occupation Model

HISTORICAL DEVELOPMENT

During the past two decades, changes in occupational therapy theories and practice have led to greater consideration of the transactional relationships between children and youth; the occupations in which they engage; and the environments in which they live, play, and learn. Although occupational therapy assessment and intervention with children and youth remains more weighted in the direction of the person, there is an increased focus on elements of the environment that influence participation in occupations (Law, 2002). Therapists acknowledge the potential therapeutic impact of the environment as well as the complex relationship between the person and environment. Models of practice in occupational therapy that have been developed over the past 20 years have incorporated these changing views of the importance of environments in determining participation (Canadian Association of Occupational Therapists [CAOT], 1997; Dunn, Brown, & McGuigan, 1994; Kielhofner, 2002). Specifically, such models have challenged occupational therapists to develop increased understanding of person-environment inter-actions and the role that environments play in both assessment and intervention.

In the early 1990s, six occupational therapists at McMaster University in Canada formed a research group to study the influence of environments on occupational perfor-mance. The group began by reviewing literature on environment-behavior theories (Law, Cooper, Stewart, Letts, Rigby, & Strong, 1994) and environmental assessments (Letts, Law, Rigby, Cooper, Stewart, & Strong, 1994). Further exploration and synthesis of these ideas led to the development of a conceptual model, the Person-Environment-Occupation (PEO) model that reflected the dynamic and transactive relationships between persons, their environments, and their occupations (Law, Cooper, Strong, Stewart, Rigby, & Letts, 1996; Strong, Rigby, Stewart, Law, Letts, & Cooper, 1999). The purpose of the model was to provide occupational therapists with increased understanding of these relationships, as well as to serve as an analytic tool for determining assessment and intervention.

Theoretical foundations for the PEO model build on concepts and assumptions from Lawton and Nahemow (1973), Csikszentmihalyi (1990), current Canadian guidelines for occupational therapy practice (CAOT, 1997), and the Canadian Occupational Performance Measure (COPM) (Law, Baptiste, Carswell, McColl, Polatajko, & Pollock, 2005). Within the PEO model, occupational performance results from the dynamic, ongoing relationship between people; their occupations and roles; and the environments in which they live, work, and play. Environments continually influence behavior as well as behavior affect-ing environments. Occupational therapy assessment and intervention need to consider all aspects of occupational performance, the child, their environment, and their desired occupation. The goal of occupational therapy services for children is to enable optimal occupational performance in those occupations identified as important by the child or youth and their family.

THEORETICAL UNDERPINNINGS

The PEO model approaches the study of occupational performance from an ecologi-cal point of view. Thus, the model is informed by environment-behavior theories, with origins in the disciplines of environmental psychology, architecture, anthropology, human geography, and social science. The ideas of environmental press developed by Lewin (1935) and need-press by Murray (1938) form the basis of an ecological approach. Environments are not passive but exert influences on persons at all times. For example, the home environment exerts an important and continual influence on a child's develop-ment and behavior. In particular, the theories of Bronfenbrenner are an essential under-pinning of the PEO model as it applies to children.

Bronfenbrenner studied human social development and the factors that influenced development as children grew. In his Ecological Systems model (1977), he describes the nature of social development of a person over his or her life span. The interdependent relationships between home, family, school, work, community, and country systems are emphasized. As Bronfenbrenner states:

> The ecology of human development involves the scientific study of the progressive mutual accommodation between an active, growing human being and the changing properties of the immediate settings in which the developing person lives, as this process is affected by relations between these settings, and by the larger contexts in which the settings are embed-ded. (1979, p. 21)

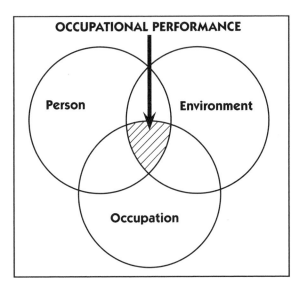

Figure 3-1. The Person-Environment-Occupation model. (Reprinted with permission of CAOT Publications ACE. From Law, M., Cooper, B., Strong, S., Stewart, D., Rigby, P., & Letts, L. [1996]. The person-environment-occupation model: A transactive approach to occupational performance. *Canadian Journal of Occupational Therapy, 63,* 9-23.)

Most recently, Bronfenbrenner has described a bioecological model of human development with relationships between developmental process, persons, context, and time affecting the lifecourse of an individual (Bronfenbrenner, 1995).

Other theorists whose concepts inform the PEO model are the work of Csikszentmihalyi (1990) and Larson and Verma (1999). These researchers have studied children's time use and experience of participating in different activities. Csikszentmihalyi (1990) has demonstrated that the relationship between the challenges of an activity and individual skills determine the activity experience. For example, if a child is just learning to play the piano, the challenges may be greater than the child's skill, leading to anxiety. Satisfaction with an activity is enhanced when there is congruence or fit between the child's skills, the demands of the activity (occupation), and the demands of the environment.

From the profession of occupational therapy, the PEO model is informed by the Canadian guidelines for client-centered practice (CAOT, 1997). In particular, the model supports the view that persons receiving occupational therapy services are partners in the therapy process. Children and their families know the occupational performance issues facing the child every day. Therefore, identification of issues for therapy intervention is best done by the child (if old enough) and his or her family. Within the PEO model, the COPM (Law, Baptiste, et al., 2005) and the Perceived Efficacy and Goal Setting System (Missiuna, Pollock, & Law, 2004) are client- and family-centered methods for occupational performance issue identification.

Overview of the Person-Environment-Occupation Model

The PEO model describes the transactional relationships between person, occupation, and environment; outlines major concepts and assumptions; and applies these ideas to an occupational therapy practice situation. The model recognizes and celebrates the complexity of performance of occupations within different environmental contexts.

Figure 3-1 illustrates the PEO model. In this Venn diagram, the three components of the model (person, environment, and occupation) are drawn as linked circles. The overlap of the three circles represents occupational performance. Figure 3-2 illustrates the PEO process through time to indicate how these factors contribute to development throughout the lifespan. In this figure, one can see how examining person, environment,

Figure 3-2. Person-Environment-Occupation relationships over the lifespan. (Reprinted with permission of CAOT Publications ACE. From Law, M., Cooper, B., Strong, S., Stewart, D., Rigby, P., & Letts, L. [1996]. The person-environment-occupation model: A transactive approach to occupational performance. *Canadian Journal of Occupational Therapy, 63,* 9-23.)

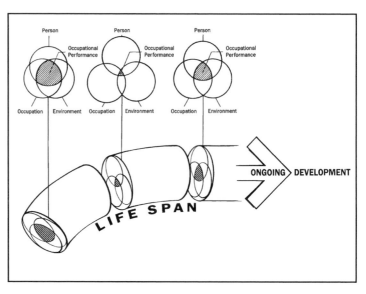

and occupation at specific points in time yields different interactions and resulting occupational performance. The characteristics of people, their occupations, and their environments are continually changing, resulting in accommodation or adaptation throughout life. In Figure 3-2, the PEO circles represent the influences on occupational performance at one point in time and the outer area within the cylinder illustrates the broader environmental context within which a person lives.

PERSON-ENVIRONMENT-OCCUPATION MODEL CONCEPTS AND ASSUMPTIONS

The key concepts and assumptions of the PEO model are as follows.

Person

Within this model, persons hold specific physical, emotional, cognitive, and spiritual characteristics (Law et al., 1996). Children hold unique personal characteristics, be it temperament, health, self-concept, skills, or personality. These characteristics interact with childhood occupations and environments to determine each experience of doing an occupation. For example, a child who is outgoing in nature may enjoy and participate frequently in the occupation of drama, while another child will enjoy a less public occupation. As children grow and develop, their occupations are influenced both by the values and beliefs of their family and those that they develop alone or with groups. Each person assumes a variety of roles throughout life—for children, their primary roles are child, learner, player, and friend. As children move into adolescence, the roles of worker and citizen develop increasing prominence. Children are also influenced by the environments in which they live, play, and learn.

Environment

Theoretical conceptualizations of the environment tend to be broad and include cultural, social, psychological, organizational, and physical components. Within the PEO model, environment is defined as "those contexts and situations which occur outside the individual and elicit responses from them" (Law, 1991, p. 175). As occupational therapists, we think of environments as including social, political, economic, institutional, physical, and cultural considerations (Law et al., 1994). Environmental locations also differ, ranging from the household to neighborhood to community and country. The environment is the context in which persons engage in occupations (Dunn et al., 1994). Environments can shape and influence behavior. For example, a play environment often elicits laughter and noisy interactions in comparison to a quieter school classroom environment.

Occupation

Occupation is defined as "groups of self-directed, functional tasks and activities in which a person engages over the lifespan" (Law et al., 1996, p. 175). Children and youth engage in occupations to meet their intrinsic needs for involvement, expression, skill development, and enjoyment. All humans have an innate need to participate in occupations (Wilcock, 1998).

Learning Activity A

Identify the person, environment, and occupation aspects of the following brief scenarios:

- Jerome is attending preschool for the first time and is expected to sit quietly during 10 minutes of circle time.
- Manuel is a 5-year-old who is playing on a soccer team but has difficulty making contact with the ball.
- Karina is a 7-year-old who now has pet care added to her daily routine.
- Mary is a single mother with two children under the age of 5 who primarily watch TV throughout the day.

OCCUPATIONAL PERFORMANCE

Within the PEO model, occupational performance is depicted as the outcome of the transactional relationships between the child, environment, and occupation. Occupational performance is experiential in nature and determined by the person who is engaged in a purposeful occupation within a specific environment. While the doing of an occupation can be observed, the experience of occupational performance is subjective in nature (McColl & Pollock, 2005).

The model recognizes that occupational performance is also determined by patterns of occupation over time. The temporal nature of PEO relationships is particularly important to consider in a developing child. The routines of occupation develop as a child grows up and continue to change over the lifespan. At each point in time, the relative influences of person, occupation, and environment may shift. For example, university students are largely influenced by other students and the educational environment in which they study. A university student who has a disability will experience more significant environmental influences on his or her ability to study effectively. As well, environments are considered to be open to change through an intervention process.

PERSON-ENVIRONMENT-OCCUPATION FIT

Within the PEO model, the three major components of person, environment, and occupation interact continually across time and space to determine occupational performance. When these components fit closely together, occupational performance is optimized (Figure 3-3). The concept of PEO fit is an important assumption of the PEO model. The basis of occupational therapy interventions rests on the belief that change in person,

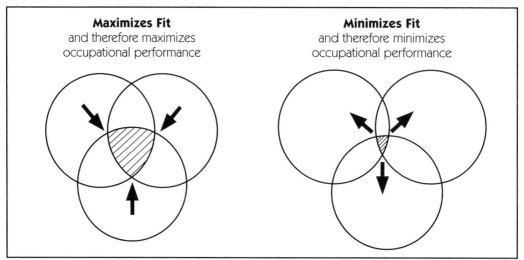

Figure 3-3. An illustration of changes to occupational performance as a consequence to changes in person, environment, and occupation fit. (Reprinted with permission of CAOT Publications ACE. From Law, M., Cooper, B., Strong, S., Stewart, D., Rigby, P., & Letts, L. [1996]. The person-environment-occupation model: A transactive approach to occupational performance. *Canadian Journal of Occupational Therapy, 63,* 9-23.)

environment, or occupation can improve PEO fit and thus improve occupational performance (Law et al., 1996). Occupational therapists can improve the enabling characteristics of the environment to improve occupation (see Figure 3-3).

The strength of the PEO model lies in the model's focus on the transactional relationship between person, occupation, and environment. The model enables therapists to analyze the relative influences of person, occupation, and environment to a child's occupational performance. Interventions can target change in the child, occupation, and/or the environment in different ways. As occupational therapists, we have multiple ways in which to facilitate occupational performance. The PEO model has undergone testing since 1990 (see Cooper & Stewart, 1997; Law et al., 1998; Stewart, Law, Rosenbaum, & Willms, 2001; Strong, 1998).

Using the Person-Environment-Occupation Model in Pediatric Occupational Therapy Practice

The use of the PEO model for occupational therapy services for children and youth has the following characteristics (Law, Baum, & Dunn, 2005):

- A family-centered approach to therapy service is used, with the child and his or her family identifying occupational performance issues for intervention.

- Interventions that target changing the child, occupation, and/or the environment are always considered.

- The model supports both individual and group interventions, as well as interventions solely focused on changing environments.

- Environmental changes can occur at each level of the environment, including home, neighborhood, community, and state/country.

- Assessment and outcome measurement within the model makes use of a broad repertoire of measures.

— SECTION II —

Application of the Person-Environment-Occupation Model

Within recent years occupational therapy literature has included the application of the PEO model in a variety of practice aspects related to intervention with children and families (Dunbar & Werner DeGrace, 2001; Hotz, Kniepmann, & Kohn, 1998; McGuire, Crowe, Law, & VanLeit, 2004). These sources offer several examples of the use of the PEO model for analysis of occupational performance issues, providing a guide to intervention planning, as well as creating a way to view interaction with the client and his or her family. In addition, application of the contextual aspects of the PEO model provides a means to consider other socioeconomic, cultural, institutional, and physical environment factors that impact daily life experiences (Strong et al., 1999).

EVALUATION AND ANALYSIS OF OCCUPATIONAL PERFORMANCE

The *Occupational Therapy Practice Framework* (American Occupational Therapy Association [AOTA], 2002) separates the evaluation process into two separate processes: the Occupational Profile and the Analysis of Occupational Performance. The Occupational Profile is an exploration of a client's barriers and needs to engagement in occupation. In addition, the client's goals are identified and the reason for referral is clarified. Identification of environmental supports and restraints for occupational performance are also identified in this initial process. The Analysis of Occupational Performance is the actual assessment of performance in occupations. Through observation as well as formal and informal assessment processes, the occupational therapist analyzes a client's performance skills, client factors, demands of the activity, and the environmental contexts that influence the performance (AOTA, 2002).

In the initial process of evaluation, the PEO model guides an occupational therapist to consider a person's skills and abilities, the tasks and activities that are meaningful to an individual, and the environments in which engagement and participation in occupations occur. The various levels of consideration in evaluation can include the individual, the individual as part of a family, or the individual in a community context. Environmental aspects that could influence occupational performance at any of these levels include cultural, institutional, physical, economic, and social factors (Law et al., 1996).

Analysis of each of the PEO aspects, in relationship to a child and his or her respective family, can provide a holistic view of a situation in the performance aspect of the evaluation process. In addition, by conceptualizing the fit between these three entities, an occupational therapist can assess the existing or potential strengths, as well as the existing or potential barriers, to optimal occupational performance. Occupational performance is the dynamic experience of engagement in meaningful activities that an individual participates in within his or her daily round of life. The greater the overlap among the three PEO spheres, the greater the opportunity for optimal occupational performance of an individual (Strong et al., 1999).

Dunbar and Werner DeGrace (2001) provide an example of the application of PEO to the evaluation process for a dyad consisting of an infant and a young mother. Lanisha (mother) and Jason (son) were seen in a neighborhood university-related health clinic. Jason was 3 months old at the time of the initial referral for a developmental assessment.

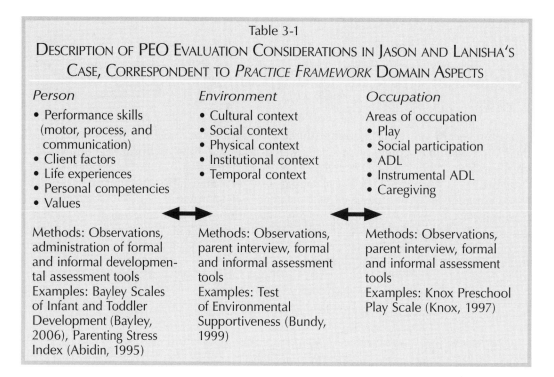

Table 3-1

DESCRIPTION OF PEO EVALUATION CONSIDERATIONS IN JASON AND LANISHA'S
CASE, CORRESPONDENT TO *PRACTICE FRAMEWORK* DOMAIN ASPECTS

Person	Environment	Occupation
• Performance skills (motor, process, and communication) • Client factors • Life experiences • Personal competencies • Values	• Cultural context • Social context • Physical context • Institutional context • Temporal context	Areas of occupation • Play • Social participation • ADL • Instrumental ADL • Caregiving
Methods: Observations, administration of formal and informal developmental assessment tools Examples: Bayley Scales of Infant and Toddler Development (Bayley, 2006), Parenting Stress Index (Abidin, 1995)	Methods: Observations, parent interview, formal and informal assessment tools Examples: Test of Environmental Supportiveness (Bundy, 1999)	Methods: Observations, parent interview, formal and informal assessment tools Examples: Knox Preschool Play Scale (Knox, 1997)

Developmental testing did not reveal any significant delays; however, he exhibited hand fisting and very limited interaction with his mother. By the second visit, following the development of a home program, Jason did not display any more developmental issues. However, his mother insisted on continued visits and stated that she needed them in order to know what to expect in child development. Lanisha felt that the interaction with the occupational therapist gave her an opportunity to understand her child's strengths and needs in more depth and she desired the additional parenting support. In this brief example, the occupational therapist was able to apply the PEO model by considering the aspects shown in Table 3-1 for both Lanisha and Jason. The arrows depict the transitive, interrelationship between the PEO areas. The PEO concepts have been illustrated in conjunction with the key areas of an occupational therapist's domain of practice.

Within a family-centered context, an analysis of the PEO can be done for the mother as well as the child, as illustrated in Table 3-1. Since the author was the treating therapist in this scenario, a more in-depth view is warranted in the discussion of the application of PEO for assessment in this case. The mother described several personal stressors (person) that impacted her ability to parent (occupation). She also described a minimally supportive home (environment) in which some of the family members did not treat her very well. She related how daycare screening and decision making (occupation) was a process that she wanted to start, but needed help in doing so. The occupational therapist realized that a point of intervention, based on the assessment and analysis process, needed to focus on the child's human environment (mother). Her needs spanned the three areas of PEO and each one of these needed to be addressed in order to optimize occupational performance in her significant role as Jason's mother. The mother's ability to successfully navigate this occupational role had a significant impact on the child's occupational performance.

Learning Activity B

1. Using the key principles of a family-centered service approach, describe the implications of these principles on the way in which occupational therapy assessment and intervention are completed.

2. PEO assessment: Using one of the chapter case examples, develop and demonstrate an assessment plan based on the PEO model. Include the following:

   - Describe the person, environment, and occupation factors that were included in the summary.
   - Identification of occupational performance issues of the person.
   - Identification of the person, environment, and occupation factors that are helping or hindering performance of the identified occupation(s).
   - Identify a minimum of two assessments that will provide more data regarding the occupational performance issues. Be able to give a rationale for your choices and identify how you prioritized these assessments. Relate to the occupational performance issues in your rationale.
   - Provide information about the clinical usefulness, reliability, validity, and the applicability of the assessment(s) under consideration.
   - Consider the applicability of the assessment to chosen practice area (e.g., cost, timing, ease of administration, etc.).
   - Provide narrative examples of how environmental factors that influence occupational performance may be discussed in an evaluation report.

3. Analysis: Analyze the person, environment, and occupation factors that are influencing a child's or adolescent's performance in the following brief scenarios. Use the analysis template provided in Tables 3-4 and 3-5 to do the analysis.

   - Jeremy, a 4-year-old child with autism, is unable to follow the routine in his childcare center, particularly during circle time.
   - Natasha, a 2-year-old, is having difficulty transitioning to any food beyond a puréed texture.
   - Karen, a teen mother, is having difficulty coordinating a schedule for childcare and her high school homework.
   - LaToya, a 15-year-old high school student, has much difficulty completing her exams due to anxiety attacks.
   - Manuel, an 18-year-old with cognitive delays who is transitioning to an independent living facility, has difficulty sequencing his breakfast preparation.

4. Analyze the PE, PO, and EO transactions influencing performance of the tasks in each scenario.

5. Describe how you would adapt the environment to enhance the occupational performance of each particular client.

6. Create an evaluation plan for a selected child from the list and his or her family to improve performance in these tasks.

Table 3-2

APPLICATION OF PEO TO TREATMENT CONSIDERATIONS WITH LANISHA

Person	Environment	Occupation
Discussions related to self-concept and personal competencies related to mothering	Collaboration with parent regarding home-made developmental toy fabrication	*Assistance in navigating daycare decision making*
Discussions related to life experiences and their relationship to mothering	Discussions related to management of less supportive family members	Assertiveness training for dealing with daycare providers Example: Role playing interactions with staff
Discussions regarding hopes/desires for Jason Discussion regarding hopes/desires for self	*Assistance in navigating daycare decision making* Example: Evaluating the institutional, cultural, and social environment	Activities related to occupations and co-occupations of mothering Example: Facilitating social play with mother and baby
Activities to improve parenting competencies Example: Asking Lanisha to share a play activity and then verbally reinforcing success	Collaboration regarding exploration of supportive neighborhood networks	**Activities to improve parenting competencies**

INTERVENTION

The information from the three aspects of PEO is brought together in a transactional structure to develop an intervention plan with a client (Strong et al., 1999). The PEO model allows the occupational therapist to intervene from multiple perspectives with children and families. Traditionally, occupational therapists working in pediatric-oriented environments have developed a more component-based orientation. Recent literature has advocated for a more holistic "top-down" perspective that allows for consideration of the environmental influence on occupational performance, as well as a more notable focus on occupational aspects (Coster, 1998). An example of a more traditional approach would be to consider a child's sensory and motor skills during treatment, without consideration of how these influence play or social participation occupations and the environments in which these aspects occur. In addition, an omission of actually engaging the child in play for play's sake or including peer interactions in treatment could also be quite limiting for children with these occupational performance concerns. The PEO model gives an opportunity for occupational therapists to intervene in occupational and environmental domains that have not been readily considered in component-oriented treatment.

In the aforementioned case, Lanisha's needs within the PEO spheres were assessed to be significant enough to warrant intervention for herself. This was done in conjunction with routine developmental check-ups for Jason. This strategy of combining interventions allowed for traditional reimbursement from the third-party payer, while continuing to address the family's needs as a whole. Table 3-2 illustrates the focus of intervention, based on the PEO model, for this mother as she struggled to understand the developmental strengths and needs of her son. The therapist's involvement in assisting Lanisha in daycare decision making impacted both the occupation and environment.

OE aspects are italicized. Activities that were provided to enhance parenting competencies in child care and fostering optimal development overlapped between the PO aspects and are bolded (see Table 3-2). This type of overlap is consistent with the frequent depiction of PEO as overlapping spheres. Intervention may need to focus on two overlapping areas at a time to optimally address the varied needs of a client.

The PEO model is useful for expanding an occupational therapist's treatment options. Instead of treating an individual irrespective of his or her family and other contextual considerations, it allows multiple perspectives for intervention. Evaluation and intervention for families will present with issues related to one or multiple aspects from a PEO perspective. Regardless of the situation, there are several aspects that will be consistent in the approach.

General PEO considerations for evaluation and treatment of a child or adolescent include the following major points (adapted from Pollock, Stewart, Law, Sahagian-Whalen, Harvey, & Toal, 1997):

1. Support a family-centered approach in which the values and perceptions of the family unit are respected.
2. Recognize the influence of culture and values in the evaluation process.
3. For evaluation and intervention of older children, support their values and perceptions as individuals as well as in the context of family and community.
4. Consider the environment as an area for evaluation, as well as a change element for intervention.
5. Appreciate the complexity of the transaction between person, environment, and occupation elements in the evaluation and treatment process.
6. Recognize the variations of perceptions regarding health, wellness, illness, and disability among individuals with special needs and their families.
7. Consider alternative roles, including consultant and advocate, for addressing issues related to occupational performance.
8. Engage in ongoing personal assessment of your own ability to listen and observe for what is meaningful to a client.

These guidelines will assist the occupational therapist in optimizing intervention for children and families by making holistic considerations for the person, environment, and the occupation.

Case Study: Application of the Person-Environment-Occupation Model

By Rhodine Thomas, BSc

INTRODUCTION

The PEO model will be used to explain an occupational therapy consultative role that was taken to analyze the participation of a child with a congenital limb deficiency on a Little League baseball team. The child lacks a right forearm and right hand and uses a prosthetic limb. The relevant supports and barriers in each domain, as well as the strategies to maximize the child's occupational performance in this sport, will be addressed.

Supports

Matt is a 10-year-old boy in Grade 4 who is motivated to play sports due to the fun and peer interaction that is involved. He also has the experience of being a member of the division-winning soccer team the summer before. This past experience, coupled with Matt's excellent communication skills and his comfort with educating others about his disability may aid his transition to another challenging sport activity. His effective communication skills were developed by doing television commercials in the past for the War Amps Association's CHAMPS program. Another "person" support is Matt's prosthetic arm, which can be easily fitted to any adaptive device that he would need to play baseball.

Barriers

Matt's prosthetic limb is also considered a barrier because it is rigid and cannot be flexed or extended to catch or throw baseballs. The finger units are fixed and immobile with only a moveable thumb unit to form a weak thumb-to-finger grasp. This grasp will be too weak to tightly grip and control the baseball or the baseball bat. The immobility of the prosthetic limb's finger units could also prevent Matt from donning a baseball glove to play baseball.

ENVIRONMENT

Supports

The Little League association offers a player development program that provides training clinics to help players develop their baseball skills. This could help Matt to learn the skills that are necessary to play on the baseball team. In addition to this, the Little League association's president indicated that there was no by-law in the Little League Canada guidelines that prohibited persons with physical impairments from participating on Little League teams. Finally, the Little League has guidelines to match a player to his or her skill level to ensure safety. Matt would be placed in a lower division if necessary, given that he has never played baseball before.

In regards to funding, an amputation association would cover the cost for any recreational adaptive devices that Matt would need to play baseball.

Barriers

One barrier that Matt faces is the time to order, be fitted with, and be trained in the use of these recreational adaptive devices. At the time of the assessment, the baseball season was only 1 month away and Matt would still need to order the appropriate devices, which take an additional 1 to 2 months to be delivered. A second timing issue was that the league was having mandatory try-out sessions as soon as the season started and since Matt had not ordered the equipment, he would be unable to participate in these try-outs. A third environmental issue was that Matt lived 30 minutes away from the baseball club and his mother would need to drive him there two to three times a week, which was not possible given that it interrupted her work schedule. A fourth issue that could affect Matt's transitioning onto this team is the level of his teammates' tolerance and understanding of his disability. This could affect Matt's comfort with the team and his motivation to play baseball.

OCCUPATION

Supports

Team positions could be rotated or altered based on a player's skill level in this Little League association. Therefore Matt could play different positions on the team after obtaining the necessary adaptive devices.

Barriers

Baseball involves several bilateral tasks such as catching, hitting, and throwing a baseball. It also requires effective gripping and control while hitting and swinging a baseball bat. Matt's ability to perform these bilateral tasks is complicated due to the rigidity of his prosthetic limb.

RECOMMENDED STRATEGIES FOR MAXIMIZING SUCCESS

Person/Occupation

1. Recommend the purchase of adaptive devices to fit to the prosthetic limb:
   a. TRS Hi-Fly Fielder (TRS Inc., Boulder, CO) (Figure 3-4) for ball catching. It is a flexible mesh pocket that allows for either forehand or backhanded catching and eliminates the need for forearm rotation.
   b. TRS Pinch Hitter (TRS Inc., Boulder, CO) (Figure 3-5). It is a flexible, rubber-based device that snaps on and off aluminum bats. The three main purposes are to control the swing of the bat, to improve swing speed, and to increase ball hitting distances.
   c. Aluminum bat, due to the fact that the TRS devices work better with these types of bats than wooden ones.
2. Enroll Matt into the player development program to develop his baseball skills with professional coaching.

Environment

1. Due to timing issues, recommend ordering the adaptive devices now to learn how to use them for the baseball season next summer.
2. In terms of transportation, recommend that Matt's mother set up carpooling rides with other children in the league.
3. In order to increase tolerance and awareness of persons with disabilities in the league, recommend that an occupational therapist meet with coaches and teammates to teach them about amputations and about the use of prosthetic devices. He or she can use coloring books and activity books to educate the children. Matt can also relate his personal experiences to his teammates to aid in the education sessions.

In summary, by using the aspects of the PEO model, the areas of support and barriers that affect Matt's ability to play on a Little League baseball team given his physical disability were highlighted. It is intended that the recommendations provided help to minimize the barriers and facilitate his transition onto the team for next summer.

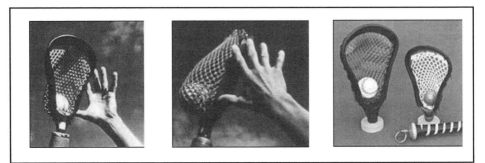

Figure 3-4. TRS Hi-Fly Fielder (TRS Inc., Boulder, CO). Length=32 cm, width (max.)=19 cm, thickness=4.5 cm, weight=314 grams, color=leather brown with black trim, age=youth/adult. (Reprinted with permission from TRS Inc. Available at http://www.oandp.com/products/trs/.)

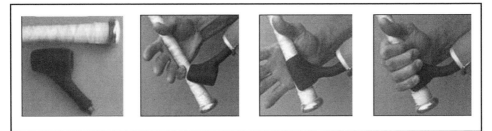

Figure 3-5. TRS Pinch Hitter (TRS Inc., Boulder, CO). Length=12 cm, width (max.)=3.8 cm, weight=98 grams, color=matte black, age=youths 8 years and older. (Reprinted with permission from TRS Inc. Available at http://www.oandp.com/products/trs/.)

Application of Person-Environment-Occupation Model to Developing and Implementing Interventions Within Organizations and Communities

CASE EXAMPLE

This example centers on improving community-based recreation services for children and youth with special needs. An occupational therapist is engaged as a consultant for a local municipality to assist the department of recreation in assessing and improving recreation services for children with special needs.

The occupational therapist begins by gathering information about the project from the Director of Recreation and the city staff/citizen committee that is guiding this process. The committee is charged by the City Council to develop an inclusion and access policy to improve the participation of children with special needs in city recreation programs (Figure 3-6).

Tables 3-3 through 3-5 also facilitate the process of PEO analysis in the community, as well as other settings.

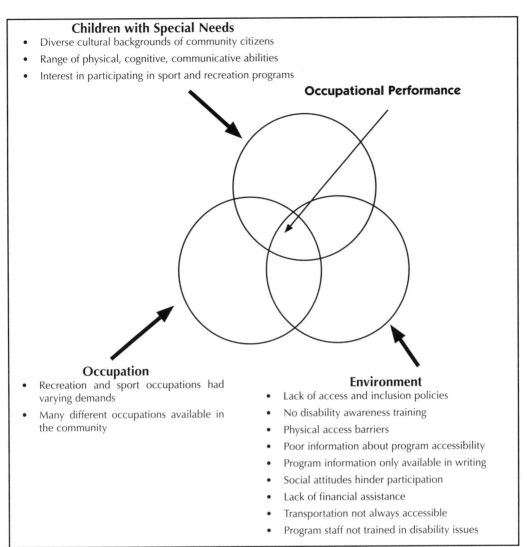

Children with Special Needs
- Diverse cultural backgrounds of community citizens
- Range of physical, cognitive, communicative abilities
- Interest in participating in sport and recreation programs

Occupational Performance

Occupation
- Recreation and sport occupations had varying demands
- Many different occupations available in the community

Environment
- Lack of access and inclusion policies
- No disability awareness training
- Physical access barriers
- Poor information about program accessibility
- Program information only available in writing
- Social attitudes hinder participation
- Lack of financial assistance
- Transportation not always accessible
- Program staff not trained in disability issues

Figure 3-6. Person-Environment-Occupation model application to organizations and community settings.

Learning Activity C

1. Identify some of the key areas of concern related to occupational performance. Example: Access to community-based recreation programs for children with disabilities.
2. Analyze the person, environment, and occupation factors that are helping or hindering success in the case example.
3. Identify other methods of data collection in each of the person, environment, and occupation areas that supported the occupational therapist's intervention in the case example.

   Example:

   Person. Methods of data collection included observations of recreation programs.

   Occupation. Methods of data collection included inventory of community recreation activities and programs.

Table 3-3

APPLICATION OF PEO TO INTERVENTION PLAN FOR THIS COMMUNITY

Person	Environment	Occupation
Recommended methods to ensure assessment of the preferences of children with special needs regarding their desired participation in sport and recreation activities within their community	Development of a municipal access and inclusion to recreation policy Development of a community-based resource group to monitor and assist with policy implementation	Provision of information and training regarding adaptation of sport and recreation activities for children with special needs
	Human resources department develop training opportunities for staff Municipality uses most complete universal access guides for building standards for recreation and sport facilities Include access symbols in all program information Produce program information in different formats Change facilities to upgrade physical access	

Person-Environment-Occupation Model and Frames of Reference

Although the PEO model is a holistic and transactive approach that is applicable to a variety of intervention situations, it is often necessary to combine the model with a frame of reference to best meet the needs of a client. As described in Chapter 1, a model enables a practitioner to view a situation from a wider lens. The "big picture" perspective is all encompassing and can create a vision for intervening from either an individual or a larger contextual perspective. However, within the "big picture" are smaller entities that need to be addressed.

Examples of these smaller entities may include performance skills and client factors. When issues in any of these areas hinder occupational performance, additional frameworks are needed. For example, when a child experiences tactile defensiveness he or she may be hindered in his or her ability to play in the sandbox. Sensory function is considered a body function and a subcategory of client factors, as defined in the *Occupational Therapy Practice Framework* (AOTA, 2002). Application of complementary frames of reference that address performance skills and client factor issues can provide the occupational therapist a means of addressing the specific needs of an individual.

Table 3-4

ANALYSIS TEMPLATE

Analysis of the child, environment, and occupation factors influencing performance

Child _____   Therapist _____

Date _____

Goal/Occupation:		
Factors that help or hinder the child to perform this occupation		
Child Help:	**Occupation** Help:	**Environment** Help:
Hinder:	Hinder:	Hinder:

Intervention: Yes _____, focus of intervention

No _____, explain why

(Adapted from Law, M., Darrah, J., Russell, D., Rosenbaum, P., Walter, S., Wilson, B., & Petrenchik, T. National Institutes of Health: $745,303, September 2005-September 2008. *Family-centred functional therapy for children with cerebral palsy.*)

Dunbar (1999) describes Sara, a 3-year-old girl who was referred to occupational therapy due to behavioral problems that were demonstrated in her preschool environment.

An outpatient evaluation utilizing a sensory history (Cook, 1991), the DeGangi-Berk Test of Sensory Integration (Berk & DeGangi, 1987), the Early Intervention Developmental Profile (Schafer & Moersch, 1981), the Knox Preschool Play Scale (Knox, 1997), parent interview, and clinical observations, revealed significant limitations in her occupational performance. Figure 3-7 illustrates the PEO aspects that were noted in the evaluation process.

The PEO model was used to gain perspective on the various aspects that influenced Sara's occupational performance, particularly in her home and school environments. Sara's mother indicated her goal for her daughter was to improve her ability to be successful in her preschool environment and to be safer in her home environment.

Together, the occupational therapist and the mother developed a plan of care that was individualized to meet the family needs. Sara's mother was willing to participate in a home program and an integrated approach with home activities and outpatient treatment was planned. Table 3-6 is a list of sample treatment aspects within the context of the three PEO domains.

Table 3-5

ANALYSIS TEMPLATE—COMPLETED

Analysis of the child, environment, and occupation factors influencing performance

Child _____   Therapist _____

Date _____

Goal/Occupation: *Feeding self with spoon*		
Factors that help or hinder the child to perform this occupation		
Child	**Occupation**	**Environment**
Help: *Determination. Self-motivated. Wants to feed self. Understands what self-feeding means. Does not want parents to help.*	Help: *Frequency of occupation with many practice opportunities. Task is typically self-motivating as feedback is instantaneous.*	Help: *Preschool setting very structured for feeding routines.*
Hinder: *Spasticity affects quality of movement in upper extremities. Grasp of spoon inconsistent. Lack of refined wrist and hand movement.*	Hinder: *Self-feeding can be messy. Type of utensils used. Parents concerned with cleanliness of child.*	Hinder: *Child easily distracted by others in same room. Positioning of child at table.*
Intervention: Yes _____, focus of intervention *Emphasize performance rather than quality of self-feeding and cleanliness. Provision of appropriate seating and feeding aids.* No _____, explain why		

(Adapted from Law, M., Darrah, J., Russell, D., Rosenbaum, P., Walter, S., Wilson, B., & Petrenchik, T. National Institutes of Health: $745,303, September 2005-September 2008. *Family-centred functional therapy for children with cerebral palsy.*)

Table 3-6 illustrates the blend of considerations within the three PEO aspects. The combined approach of the model and frames of reference enables an occupational therapist to be creative in optimizing the evaluation and treatment families. In this particular case, Sara made remarkable gains and was able to complete play tasks, decrease adverse reactions in social situations, and self-organize in more challenging situations. This was done with combining aspects of the Sensory Integration (refer to Chapter 2) and Psychosocial frames of reference with the overarching considerations of the person, environment, and occupation.

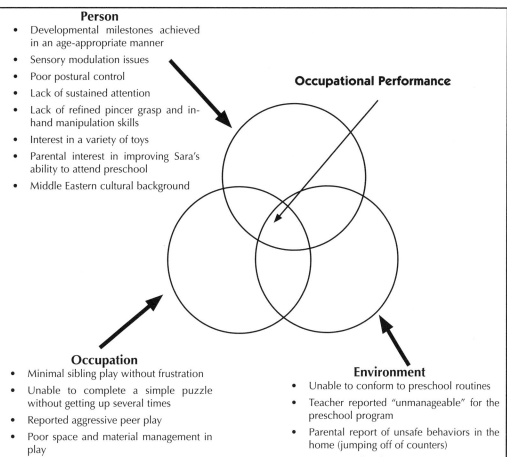

Person
- Developmental milestones achieved in an age-appropriate manner
- Sensory modulation issues
- Poor postural control
- Lack of sustained attention
- Lack of refined pincer grasp and in-hand manipulation skills
- Interest in a variety of toys
- Parental interest in improving Sara's ability to attend preschool
- Middle Eastern cultural background

Occupational Performance

Occupation
- Minimal sibling play without frustration
- Unable to complete a simple puzzle without getting up several times
- Reported aggressive peer play
- Poor space and material management in play

Environment
- Unable to conform to preschool routines
- Teacher reported "unmanageable" for the preschool program
- Parental report of unsafe behaviors in the home (jumping off of counters)
- Supportive family

Figure 3-7. Person-Environment-Occupation model evaluation.

Table 3-6

TREATMENT FOCUS EXAMPLES

Person	*Environment*	*Occupation*
Sensory integration for underresponsive vestibular system, sequencing, organization, etc.	Collaboration with parent regarding home strategies	Graded age-appropriate play activities
	Development of a community playground program	Sibling play activities
Behavioral management strategies	Structuring treatment space to increase organized behavior	Social participation activities

Considerations of the Psychosocial frame of reference in conjunction with the PEO model are warranted in this case, due to Sara's difficulty with self-control in her home and school environment and an immediate need to intervene. The Psychosocial frame of reference is critical to consider for children who exhibit sensory processing issues that may impact their relationships with peers and family (Olson, 1999). This frame of reference focuses on intervention that promotes optimal interpersonal relationships and supportive coping strategies, as well as play interests and skills. In addition, the Psychosocial frame of reference integrates the assessment of environmental supports for optimal occupational performance (Olson, 1999). This integrates well with the three overlapping areas of the PEO model by considering the person (coping abilities), environment (home, community, and school supports and barriers), as well as the occupation (play skills).

Postulates regarding change within the Psychosocial frame of reference are geared toward interventions that will enhance optimal performance in the aforementioned areas. For instance, in Sara's case she had difficulty interacting successfully with her peers. If the therapist assisted Sara in developing basic social skills needed to play with other children, then positive peer interactions will tend to increase over time.

Strong and colleagues (1999) describe another case involving a 9-year-old by the name of Karen. Karen was diagnosed with spastic diplegia and had been referred for school-based occupational therapy services. The assessment was done from a PEO perspective with the following resulting concerns in occupational performance:

1. Person
   - Motor planning difficulties
   - Lack of initiative to seek help
2. Environment
   - Teacher helping others but not Karen
3. Occupation
   - Slow pace of writing
   - Difficulty with copying from the blackboard

The authors identify a poor fit between Karen's abilities (P) and the teacher's lack of assistance (E), as well as between Karen's competency level (P) and the writing tasks given in the classroom (O). Intervention strategies that were recommended included the education of school staff, accommodations for school work, and empowering Karen with problem-solving strategies (Strong et al., 1999).

Considerations of combining frames of reference in this particular example will be made to further illustrate the feasibility of an integrated approach. Children with cerebral palsy often demonstrate issues related to visual perceptual and biomechanical areas of function due to neurological impairments (Howle, 2002). Addressing these types of concerns from a frame of reference standpoint, in conjunction with the broader perspective of PEO, is advantageous.

The Visual Information Analysis (Todd, 1999) incorporates areas related to the cognitive skills used for receiving and organizing visual information from the surrounding environment. The visual information is then integrated with other senses and experiences in order to participate in occupations. The evaluation of visual attention, visual memory, and visual discrimination provides a school-based occupational therapist with valuable information related to "person" within the context of educational activities, such as handwriting.

The biomechanical frame of reference is often considered for children with cerebral palsy as well, due to the resulting neuromuscular and musculoskeletal issues that accompany the diagnosis. This frame of reference is applied when an individual cannot independently maintain his or her posture or alignment and external supports are required to enhance occupational performance (Colangelo, 1999). By reducing the demands of gravity and improving skilled function through the use of adequate supports, an individual can improve his or her participation in everyday experiences. For instance, seating supports may be evaluated in the case of a child who is having difficulty with handwriting at his or her desk. In addition, the type of writing utensil may need to be changed to offer grip support. An occupational therapist can feasibly integrate the use of Neurodevelopmental Treatment to facilitate improved posture and alignment through handling at key points of control. These combined approaches address the person issues as well as the environmental issues that are pertinent for optimal occupational performance for a variety of children with neuromuscular issues.

Frames of reference delineate a specific area of practice (Mosey, 1981). They are applicable for managing problems within a designated area of concern. Quite often, this is related to person aspects, such as neurodevelopmental functioning, behavioral management, or biomechanical issues. Although necessary for optimal intervention in these specific areas, they do not always address the broader perspective of family or environment. In addition, critical aspects such as institutional, cultural, and even sociopolitical aspects of client functioning are not addressed in most frames of reference. These limitations necessitate a consideration of a combined approach of integrating a model or models with frames of reference. The brief cases illustrate the benefits of this unique approach.

Learning Activity D

1. Using the same brief scenarios in Learning Activity A, describe how you would adapt the environment to enhance the occupational performance of each client.

2. Describe how you would provide intervention to address person factors hindering performance in order to enhance the occupational performance of this particular client.

3. Describe how you would change the task to enhance the occupational performance of each client.

The PEO model gives occupational therapists a way to view children and their families from a holistic perspective. By emphasizing analysis of all three key aspects, treatment planning and intervention may be optimized to meet the needs of individuals within their contexts of everyday living. Application of the PEO model to a variety of settings is possible due to the generic nature of assessing the person, environment, and occupation aspects in any situation regardless of occupational need, disability, or environmental issue. Family-centered and occupation-centered care can only be enhanced by considering the whole experience of individuals who we continue to interact with in our practices on a daily basis.

References

Abidin, R. R. (1995). *Parenting Stress Index* (3rd ed.). Odessa, FL: Psychological Assessment Resources, Inc.

American Occupational Therapy Association. (2002). Occupational therapy practice framework: Domain and process. *American Journal of Occupational Therapy, 56,* 609-639.

Bayley, N. (2006). *Bayley Scales of Infant and Toddler Development (Bayley-III)* (3rd ed.). San Antonio, TX: Harcourt Assessment Inc.

Berk, R. A., & DeGangi, G. A. (1987). *DeGangi-Berk Test of Sensory Integration manual.* Los Angeles: Western Psychological Services.

Bronfenbrenner, U. (1977). Toward an experimental ecology of human development. *American Psychologist, 32,* 513-531.

Bronfenbrenner, U. (1979). *The ecology of human development.* Cambridge, MA: Harvard University Press.

Bronfenbrenner, U. (1995). The bioecological model from a life course perspective: Reflections of a participant observer. In P. Moen, G. H. Elder, & K. Luscher (Eds.), *Examining lives in context: Perspectives on the ecology of human development* (pp. 599-618). Washington, DC: American Psychological Association.

Bundy, A. C. (1999). *Test of Environmental Supportiveness.* Ft. Collins, CO: Colorado State University.

Canadian Association of Occupational Therapists. (1997). *Enabling occupation: An occupational therapy perspective.* Ottawa, Ontario, Canada: CAOT Publications ACE.

Colangelo, C. A. (1999). Biomechanical frame of reference. In P. Kramer & J. Hinojosa (Eds.), *Frames of reference in pediatric occupational therapy* (2nd ed., pp. 257-322). Baltimore: Lippincott, Williams & Wilkins.

Cook, D. G. (1991). The assessment process. In W. Dunn (Ed.), *Pediatric occupational therapy: Facilitating effective service provision* (pp. 58-60). Thorofare, NJ: SLACK Incorporated.

Cooper, B., & Stewart, D. (1997). The effect of a transfer device in the homes of elderly women. *Physical and Occupational Therapy in Geriatrics, 15,* 61-77.

Coster, W. (1998). Occupation-centered assessment of children. *American Journal of Occupational Therapy, 52,* 337-344.

Csikszentmihalyi, M. (1990). *Flow: The psychology of optimal experience.* New York: Harper & Row.

Dunbar, S. B. (1999). A child's occupational performance: Considerations of sensory processing and family context. *American Journal of Occupational Therapy, 53,* 231-235.

Dunbar, S. B., & Werner DeGrace, B. (2001). Occupational therapy models for today's practice with children and families. *OT Practice, 6*(21), 15-18.

Dunn, W., Brown, C., & McGuigan, A. (1994). The ecology of human performance: A framework for considering the effect of context. *American Journal of Occupational Therapy, 48,* 595-607.

Hotz, M., Kniepmann, K., & Kohn, L. (1998). Occupational therapy in pediatric lead exposure prevention. *American Journal of Occupational Therapy, 52*(1), 53-59.

Howle, J. (2002). *Neuro-developmental treatment approach: Theoretical foundations and principles of clinical practice.* Laguna Beach, CA: NeuroDevelopmental Treatment Association.

Kielhofner, G. (2002). *A model of human occupation: Theory and application.* Hagerstown, MD: Lippincott, Williams & Wilkins.

Knox, S. (1997). Development and current use of the Knox Preschool Play Scale. In L. D. Parham & L. S. Fazio (Eds.), *Play in occupational therapy for children* (pp. 35-51). St. Louis, MO: Mosby-Year Book.

Larson, R. W., & Verma, S. (1999). How children and adolescents spend time across the world: Work, play, and developmental opportunities. *Psychological Bulletin, 125,* 701-736.

Law, M. (1991). The environment: A focus for occupational therapy. *Canadian Journal of Occupational Therapy, 58,* 171-179.

Law, M. (2002). Participation in the occupations of everyday life. *American Journal of Occupational Therapy, 56,* 640-649.

Law, M., Baptiste, S., Carswell, A., McColl, M., Polatajko, H., & Pollock, N. (2005). *Canadian Occupational Performance Measure* (4th ed.). Ottawa, Ontario, Canada: CAOT Publications.

Law, M., Baum, C., & Dunn, W. (2005). *Measuring occupational performance* (2nd ed.). Thorofare, NJ: SLACK Incorporated.

Law, M., Cooper, B., Stewart, D., Letts, L., Rigby, P., & Strong, S. (1994). Person-environment relations. *Work, 4,* 228-238.

Law, M., Cooper, B., Strong, S., Stewart, D., Rigby, P., & Letts, L. (1996). The person-environment-occupation model: A transactive approach to occupational performance. *Canadian Journal of Occupational Therapy, 63,* 9-23.

Law, M., Darrah, J., Rosenbaum, P., Pollock, N., King, G., Russell, D., Palisano, R., Harris, S., Walter, S., Armstrong, R., & Watt, J. (1998). Family-centred functional therapy for children with cerebral palsy: An emerging practice model. *Physical and Occupational Therapy in Pediatrics, 18,* 83-102.

Lawton, M., & Nahemow, L. (1973). An ecological theory of adaptive behavior and ageing. In C. Eisdorfer & M. Lawton (Eds.), *The psychology of adult development and ageing* (pp. 657-667). Washington, DC: American Psychological Association.

Letts, L., Law, M., Rigby, P., Cooper, B., Stewart, D., & Strong, S. (1994). Person-environment assessments in occupational therapy. *American Journal of Occupational Therapy, 48,* 608-618.

Lewin, K. (1935). *Dynamic theory of personality.* New York: McGraw Hill.

McGuire, B., Crowe, T., Law, M., & VanLeit, B. (2004). Mothers of children with disabilities: Occupational concerns and solutions. *Occupational Therapy Journal of Research, 24,* 54-63.

McColl, M., & Pollock, N. (2005). Measuring occupational performance using a client-centered perspective. In M. Law, C. Baum, & W. Dunn (Eds.), *Measuring occupational performance: A guide to best practice* (2nd ed.). Thorofare, NJ: SLACK Incorporated.

Missiuna, C., Pollock, N., & Law, M. (2004). *Perceived Efficacy and Goal Setting system (PEGS).* San Antonio, TX: Psychological Corp.

Mosey, A. C. (1981). *Occupational therapy: Configuration of a profession.* New York: Raven Press.

Murray, H. (1938). *Explorations in personality.* New York: Oxford.

Olson, L. J. (1999). Psychosocial frame of reference. In P. Kramer & J. Hinojosa (Eds.), *Frames of reference in pediatric occupational therapy* (2nd ed., pp. 323-376). Baltimore: Lippincott, Williams & Wilkins.

Pollock, N., Stewart, D., Law, M., Sahagian-Whalen, S., Harvey, S., & Toal, C. (1997). The meaning of play for young people with physical disabilities. *Canadian Journal of Occupational Therapy, 64,* 25-31.

Schafer, D. S., & Moersch, M. S. (1981). *Developmental programming for infants and young children* (3rd ed., Rev.). Ann Arbor, MI: University of Michigan Press.

Stewart, D., Law, M., Rosenbaum, P., & Willms, D. (2001). A quantitative study of the transition to adulthood for youth with physical disabilities. *Physical and Occupational Therapy in Pediatrics, 21,* 3-22.

Strong, S. (1998). Meaningful work in supportive environments. *American Journal of Occupational Therapy, 52,* 31-38.

Strong, S., Rigby, P., Stewart, D., Law, M., Letts, L., & Cooper, B. (1999). Application of the person-environment-occupation model: A practical tool. *Canadian Journal of Occupational Therapy, 66,* 122-133.

Todd, V. R. (1999). Visual information analysis: Frame of reference for visual perception. In P. Kramer & J. Hinojosa (Eds.), *Frames of reference in pediatric occupational therapy* (2nd ed., pp. 205-256). Baltimore: Lippincott, Williams & Wilkins.

Wilcock, A. A. (1998). Reflections on doing, being and becoming. *Canadian Journal of Occupational Therapy, 65,* 248-257.

Application of the Model of Human Occupation to Children and Family Interventions

Jessica M. Kramer, MS, OTR/L
Patricia Bowyer, EdD, OTR/L, BCN

Learning Objectives

At the end of this chapter, the reader will be able to:

- Understand and define concepts from the Model of Human Occupation (MOHO) as they apply to children.
- Apply MOHO concepts to the occupational therapy process of evaluation, intervention, and outcome as illustrated through case studies.
- Describe MOHO-based pediatric assessments and identify the appropriate client populations and settings for assessment administration.
- Apply clinical questions to implement MOHO therapeutic reasoning.
- Identify literature that supports evidence-based application of MOHO with children and adolescents.

— Section I —

Introduction

A young child rolls over toward the sound of music and begins to play with a music toy. A teenager "acts up" in math class and gets sent to the office to avoid completing her assignment. A child grows up in a loving home, yet the family cannot seem to implement a routine to support the practice of self-care skills. Engagement in these occupations is influenced by many factors: the individuals' performance skills, the demands of the activity, and the context those activities are performed within. How can an occupational therapist identify what factors are impacting successful participation in occupation?

Using a theory that explains how and why people participate in occupations can help occupational therapists identify factors that interfere or support participation in occupations. Applying that theory to the occupational therapy process of evaluation, intervention, and outcome assessment facilitates a therapeutic reasoning process that supports best practice (American Occupational Therapy Association [AOTA], 2002). Implementing strategies based on an empirically sound theory and utilizing psychometrically sound assessments align occupational therapists with the profession's call for evidence-based practice. The Model of Human Occupation (MOHO) (Kielhofner, 2007) is one such practice model that is well researched, has developed tools for application, and has been successfully used with children, youth, and their families.

MOHO explains what drives a person to participate in selected occupations (volition), how a person organizes his or her life using routines and roles (habituation), and how a person experiences his or her world through his or her body (performance capacity). These personal characteristics interact within the environment, which can then support or constrain participation in occupation. Over time, a person's interaction with his or her world impacts his or her sense of occupational competence and occupational identity, resulting in successful or problematic occupational adaptation. This chapter will review the basic MOHO concepts, discuss participation and occupational adaptation, introduce the process of therapeutic reasoning using the model, and present a summary of developed tools and strategies that can be used to incorporate MOHO into clinical practice alongside other frames of reference. It should be recognized that this chapter only represents an introduction to what is a highly developed model of practice with a substantial evidence base and many resources for implementation. Therapists who wish to use this model should become familiar with *A Model of Human Occupation: Theory and Application* (Kielhofner, 2007) and with resources available at the MOHO website (www.moho.uic. edu).

Basic Concepts of the Model of Human Occupation

VOLITION

Motivation, inspiration, drive, and enthusiasm are some words that are used when considering a person's desire to participate in certain occupations. Humans have a biological mandate to be active (Kielhofner, 2007). This drive for occupation, or volition, is influenced by:

- An individual's sense of personal effectiveness while performing an activity (personal causation)
- The importance and worth attached to that activity (values)
- Enjoyment and satisfaction from engaging in that activity (interests)

Personal Causation

Personal causation is one's sense of competence and effectiveness while engaged in occupations and interacting with the environment. This sense of self shapes the interpretation of our experiences and guides future choices (Kielhofner, 2007). Personal causation is comprised of two dimensions: a sense of personal capacity and of self-efficacy.

A child's sense of *personal capacity* is related to his or her awareness of his or her capabilities to engage in activities he or she finds interesting and valuable. One child may excel in sports, another may consider him- or herself "musical," while another may feel he or she makes new friends easily. Children's perceptions of their capacity guides their activity choices as they are more likely to participate in activities they feel competent doing and more likely to avoid activities that threaten failure. A child who is able to pump his or her legs and upper body in a coordinated fashion in order to swing may feel a stronger sense of capacity for playing on the playground than a child with motor planning difficulties. A student who is unable to write at a high rate of speed may not feel a sense of personal capacity for taking notes in class, and therefore may avoid participation in class.

When a child feels that he or she is in control and able to use his or her capacities to achieve a desired outcome, a sense of self-efficacy is developed. Conversely, if a child believes that his or her actions cannot produce desired outcomes, he or she will have little incentive to actively engage with his or her world (Bandura, Barbaranelli, Caprara, & Pastorelli, 1996).

Personal causation is gradually built through continued accomplishments, a growing sense of control, and an increased belief in the ability to learn new tasks. A child who is comfortable rolling over will be motivated to explore the environment. A student who experiences success manipulating small toys may continue working on learning to tie his or her shoelaces. A child who enjoys playing games with familiar peers may feel comfortable initiating interactions with someone new. Personal causation is something felt internally, resulting in observable behaviors and forms of engagement in occupation; children and youth do not need to articulate personal causation into words. A child who feels competent and efficacious in an activity will seek out new challenges, while a child who feels a loss of control and a low sense of capacity will avoid new activities.

Values

Shaped by culture and context, values define what is important and meaningful for an individual who belongs to a certain family, community, society, and culture (Kielhofner, 2007). Values result from internalized convictions and are associated with a sense of obligation. These internalized personal convictions define what matters to a child and may also be a reflection of what matters to other important people in his or her life. A teenager whose parents have been successful through "hard work" yet have a limited education may not value school attendance and good grades. A mother whose culture values interdependence may enjoy completing her child's self-care rather than encouraging the child's "independence." In addition, commitment to a set of values requires a set of actions that are believed to be consistent to those values. This sense of obligation leads children and their caregivers to make decisions and engage in occupations that are aligned with the strong emotions related to their values. A child who wants to please authority figures such as parents or teachers may avoid breaking the rules in order to gain approval, while a youth may decide to volunteer in a soup kitchen as his or her beliefs about the importance of community service grow.

Just as culture and context shape personal and familial values, society's beliefs and values about disability and impairment influence how children with disabilities and their families view themselves and their situation. Traditionally, disability and impairment have been considered "a problem" (Linton, 1998, p. 137), abnormal (Swain, Finkelstein, French, & Oliver, 1993), or a "personal tragedy" (Oliver, 1996, p. 32). However, there is a growing disability pride movement that challenges these views of disability and calls for the disability values of interdependence, human community, personal connection, and self-determination (Gill, 1997; Longmore, 2003; Shapiro, 1993; Wehmeyer, Kelchner, & Richards, 1996). Occupational therapists should be aware of their own values and attitudes about impairment, and reflect how their beliefs and actions can influence the way clients and their families think about disability. Therapists can also support children and families in their own exploration of values and beliefs related to disability and facilitate a sense of community by introducing them to other families experiencing similar situations in informal gatherings or through organized local or national advocacy groups.

Interests

When participation in occupations is pleasurable and satisfying, children develop interests (Kielhofner, 2007). Sensory pleasure, personal fulfillment, and pride are just some ways children come to enjoy certain activities. The enjoyment a child feels when participating in an activity will influence future participation choices. A child who enjoys climbing on the playground may gravitate toward gymnastics, and a child with limited mobility who discovers freedom of movement in the water may be more likely to choose swimming activities in the future. Over time, as a result of both natural dispositions and positive experiences, a pattern of interests begins to reflect the unique preferences of an individual: a young athlete may spend the year participating on soccer and basketball teams, while a budding artist attends painting and violin lessons.

Learning Activity A

Identify and define the MOHO concepts and subconcepts that describe children's motivation for occupation.

THE VOLITIONAL PROCESS

Personal causation, interests, and values intersect to produce the thoughts and feelings children have about themselves and their world. Through the dynamic and ongoing volitional process of anticipating, choosing, experiencing, and interpreting participation in certain occupations, children's thoughts and feelings about themselves as a volitional actor begin to unfold (Kielhofner, 2007). When anticipating an activity, a child imagines what participation in that activity would be like based on past experiences, interests, and his or her sense of capacity and efficacy. This anticipation prepares a child to make a choice on whether or not he or she should engage in an activity. A child may be making an activity choice (e.g., studying vs. playing video games with friends) or an occupational choice (e.g., college vs. vocational training), but both choices are influenced in complex ways by a child's volition. The experience that results from the choice influences a child's sense of volition: did he or she find the activity fun, did he or she feel successful, did the activity match his or her convictions? This interpretation supports the development of a thought, feeling, or idea about him- or herself or the occupation, which then influences the way a future occupation is anticipated. It is through this volitional process that children make occupational choices and develop their sense of personal causation, range of interests, and values.

Learning Activity B

Identify the four phases of the volitional process.

Case Study #1: Volition

By Joan Gibbons, OTR/L

A ROUGH START

Dru is a 5-year-old African American boy who was born at 28 weeks gestation in a large urban community. His birth weight was 809 grams. As a result of his premature birth he had severe broncopulmonary dysplagia and gastro-esophageal reflux. Dru underwent a G-tube placement at 10 months, and due to extended time on a ventilator he required the placement of a tracheotomy shortly thereafter. Other medical concerns included retinopathy of prematurity and right eye esotropia. At the age of 13 months he was diagnosed with failure to thrive. Following an initial 13-month neonatal hospitalization, he was transferred to a children's hospital where his family received training for home health care and ventilator care. At that time he caught pneumonia and had to return to the hospital again. Once discharged to home, Dru immediately began to receive home nursing care, occupational therapy, physical therapy, and speech therapy through an early intervention program.

During infancy, Dru's right eye esotropia impacted his ability to sustain visual attention during activities such as reaching or attending to purposeful play activities. With the concerted assistance of the therapists in the home environment, along with his family's support, Dru walked at age 18 months.

At age 2.5 years, Dru developed a cyst in his right ear that required surgery and eventual prosthetic ear placement. At that time a tube was placed in his left ear as well. Mom shared that for nearly an entire year following the placement of the prosthetic ear, Dru lost vocal language skills and relied on communicating with gestures.

At age 3.5, with a language skill equivalent of 15 to 18 months, Dru began to attend outpatient speech therapy. At age 4 he began to receive occupational therapy and speech therapy in school, with removal of his trach occurring at nearly the same time. By age 4, Dru's global developmental was equivalent to a typically developing 2-year-old. His multiple pneumothoraces and recurring respiratory infections required intermittent ventilation and hospital admissions. At age 5 he was diagnosed with asthma.

CLINICAL OBSERVATIONS

In the first year of his life, Dru showed evidence of significant sensory processing issues. Vestibular processing issues included difficulty assuming positions against gravity, including lifting his head in prone and maintaining a seated position. He had difficulty using two hands for play, self-care, and reaching. Difficulties with vestibular-ocular and vestibular-auditory processing secondary to his medical conditions resulted in delayed information processing.

Signs of proprioceptive processing difficulties also surfaced. Dru had an elevated and retracted shoulder girdle, excessive extensor posturing of his neck and trunk, and subsequent resistance to positions of flexion. He lacked the ability to co-contract his muscles to gain stability in sitting and standing, and his movements lacked fluidity.

Dru also demonstrated difficulties with tactile processing. This was marked by significant oral aversion during feeding and difficulty organizing and sustaining a sucking pattern. Attempts to provide cheek support or tactile input to the face or oral cavity were met with grimacing and refusal behaviors. Decreased endurance and tactile defensiveness to textures also limited his oral intake.

A Super Trooper

The staff working with Dru was amazed at his upbeat, smiling, and playful disposition, in spite of numerous medical complications and periods of acute illness. When interviewing Dru's mother, she stated that the only time he did not appear motivated was during acute phases of illness. She shared that Dru has always been motivated to play and was always able to make choices regarding toy preferences. When asked what she thought Dru valued, she stated that he has always valued the personal attention of both she and Dru's maternal grandmother.

Dru's mother and grandmother implemented a routine that supports Dru's interests and values. Dru's mother reported that Dru had preferences for what to eat for breakfast, that he enjoyed watching the meal being prepared, and has always watched a preferred television program immediately following breakfast. Dru engages in play activities throughout the day whether residing with mom or maternal grandmother, and his preferences for activities differ according to which environment he is playing within.

In a recent interview, Dru's mother shared some of her stress and frustrations in meeting Dru's constant medical needs.

"I feel like Dru's issues have become more important than anything else, even though there are other important things I have to take care of. I feel overwhelmed, alone, and sometimes I feel like I am not doing enough to help my son."

Dru's mother had additional sources of stress in her daily life. She had to commute to a job that was a great distance from her son and the hospital that provided his care, which made her days long and limited her ability to be immediately available to help Dru. Dru's mother also described his father's involvement as "spotty" throughout the course of Dru's life. She attributes his father's excuses for not being involved and his lack of attentiveness to his inability to deal with his emotions regarding his Dru's medical and developmental difficulties.

Selection of a Therapy Framework

It was evident that successful occupational therapy intervention would utilize multiple models and frames of reference due to the scope of Dru's needs. The sensory integration (SI) frame of reference could address Dru's sensory processing difficulties, and was appropriate given Dru's medical history and diagnosis. It also became evident that the MOHO could be used to understand Dru's motivation, routines, and occupational participation. In addition, MOHO helped the occupational therapist gain a better perspective of how Dru's mother's values and habits both supported Dru's participation and were impacted by her son's medical condition. Subsequently, this resulted in the occupational therapist meeting both Dru's and his mother's needs.

New Role of Student

When Dru reached school age and was enrolled in a preschool program, Dru's sensory processing difficulties made it hard for him to meet the demands of the preschool environment. Decreased use of both hands during school and self-care tasks, problems sequencing the steps to familiar activities, and tentativeness when playing on the playground or with other children began to interfere with Dru's participation in his preschool program and role as a "student."

Proximal weakness, difficulty modulating the force of movements, uncoordinated prehension and hand manipulation, and difficulty planning novel movements—all stemming from difficulties with proprioceptive processing—continued to impact Dru's role performance. Mild esotropia in the right eye also interfered with his visual attention to tasks. Tactile processing concerns persisted as well. These included difficulty localizing touch and Dru's continued reluctance to explore new textures either with his hands or when encouraged to try new foods.

As a result of these difficulties, Dru often became frustrated and angry. However, he had difficulty communicating his feelings, which often led to "acting out" behavior. The occupational therapist was instrumental in helping Dru's mother and teacher understand that Dru's behaviors were related to his sensory processing difficulties and required support rather than punishment. As a result, Dru's mother, teachers, and therapists began to encourage Dru to use gestures and words to express his feelings. However, they all observed that Dru began to withdraw during school activities and continued to avoid interacting with other children.

INTERVENTION

The occupational therapy intervention for Dru has been based on both the SI frame of reference and MOHO. SI intervention typically uses play-oriented opportunities that are appealing to the child to introduce sensory experiences that facilitate processing for optimal functioning. This tenant of SI was strengthened by the simultaneous application of MOHO. The therapist wanted to re-capture Dru's strong sense of motivation that he had previously demonstrated in more familiar and less challenging environments. In order to better understand Dru's sense of volition, the therapist completed a Pediatric Volitional Questionnaire (PVQ) in a familiar and comfortable environment (Dru's grandmother's house) as well as an unfamiliar and more demanding environment (the therapy gym) (Figure 4-1).

At Dru's grandmother's house, a familiar and comfortable environment, Dru was familiar with environment specific activities and games—he often used his imagination and even modified familiar activities (such as moving around a plastic basketball hoop) to make them "silly" and more challenging. However, Dru's grandmother and Dru made efforts to make the home familiar and easier to access considering his specific processing difficulties. Dru's grandmother was a supportive playmate, and he depended on her to help him with problem solving and keeping on task with the activity until it was over, including the clean-up of toys and other materials. Comparing the PVQ ratings from Dru's grandmother's house with the ratings completed during the therapy session revealed that Dru was clearly having difficulties with his volition at therapy. To support Dru's volition in therapy, the therapeutic environment would be set up in a manner similar to Dru's grandmother's home environment. The therapist decided to implement a familiar therapy routine that would enable Dru to anticipate the next activity. Dru would then be able to more actively participate in the organization and set-up of the necessary objects needed for each activity. The therapist also decided to model her behavior off of Dru's grandmother—a playmate who encouraged and supported Dru to keep trying and explore alternatives when he encountered challenges in his play.

With respect to Dru's SI processing, when the occupational therapist observed Dru's sensory seeking and sensory avoiding behaviors in each of the SI domains, it was found that he sought proprioceptive input, showed a combination of seek and avoidance behaviors in the realm of tactile processing, and demonstrated avoidance behavior in response to vestibular stimulation due to hypersensitivity. During therapy sessions, Dru sought movement but was reluctant to be on moving equipment, such as swings and trampolines, with his feet off the ground. Contributing to this fear was his esotropia, which caused insecurity during movement.

During therapy sessions, movement was provided beginning with anterior-posterior movements, progressing to provision of lateral movements, and lastly to provision of

Session I Setting: Grandmother's house													
S	S	S	S	S	S	S	S	S	S	S	S	S	S
I	I	I	I	I	I	I	I	I	I	I	I	I	I
H	H	H	H	H	H	H	H	H	H	H	H	H	H
P	P	P	P	P	P	P	P	P	P	P	P	P	P
Shows Curiosity	Initiates Actions	Task-Directed	Shows Preferences	Tries New Things	Stays Engaged	Expresses Mastery Pleasure	Tries to Solve Problems	Tries to Produce Effects	Practices Skill	Seeks Challenges	Modifies Environment	Pursues Activity to Completion	Uses Imagination
Session II Setting: Therapy gym, outpatient													
S	S	S	S	S	S	S	S	S	S	S	S	S	S
I	I	I	I	I	I	I	I	I	I	I	I	I	I
H	H	H	H	H	H	H	H	H	H	H	H	H	H
P	P	P	P	P	P	P	P	P	P	P	P	P	P

PVQ Rating Scale: S=spontaneous, I=involved, H=hesitant, P=passive.

Figure 4-1. Dru's ratings on the PVQ. (Reprinted with permission from the MOHO Clearinghouse, Dept. of Occupational Therapy, University of Illinois at Chicago.)

rotary movements. Weight-bearing activities against gravity, such as lying on the platform swing, were also utilized. Toys and props that provided tactile stimulation were also provided to Dru for imaginative play. Tactile mediums such as putty and beans were also used to facilitate bilateral hand play, some of which afforded hand strengthening. Heavy work activities within the context of play were offered to help Dru strengthen his muscles and to facilitate improved body awareness.

A picture was taken of Dru doing each of these sensory-based activities, and the pictures were used to generate an activity schedule at the beginning of each session. Dru selected the activities pictured and placed them in the order he preferred. Immediately, Dru was able to demonstrate preferences, consistently wanting to choose certain activities (such as using the body sock) and avoiding others (the barrel swing). However, he was required to fill each activity slot with a different activity. This required Dru to explore new sensory activities that he otherwise would have avoided. With the therapist as a supportive playmate, Dru began to express signs of enjoyment such as clapping, laughing, and increased social interaction even during the activities he found more challenging.

DRU AND HIS FAMILY TODAY

Dru is now in a half-day school program, and he attends a YMCA after school program. He is taking medication to assist with attention difficulties and is receiving occupational therapy and speech therapy at school. The outpatient occupational therapist coordinated with the day school occupational therapist and other staff to help them set up a comfortable and more predictable environment for Dru, which includes the use of a picture schedule. Dru is also demonstrating improvements in his sensory processing and is less resistant to vestibular and tactile input, but he continues to receive outpatient occupational therapy for SI intervention.

Dru's mother is now eligible to receive respite care in the home and is also on a waiver program that allows her to pay her mother for assisting in Dru's care. As a result, Dru's mother has completed additional schooling and is looking for a job closer to home. She also takes time for herself each week away, going to the beauty shop or to a movie with a friend. As a result, she feels that she is providing for Dru without compromising her own needs. Recently, Dru's father has also become more consistently involved with Dru, inviting him for overnights on the weekend to his home and occasionally taking him to therapy sessions when his mother is working. This additional involvement has enabled Dru's mother and grandmother to continue their intense level of support for Dru and his development.

Case Study #1 Learning Activity

1. What types of activities does Dru value and have interest in, and how do they impact his participation at home, school, and in therapy?

2. Apply the volitional process to Dru's engagement in the new role of being a student.
   - How does he experience school activities?
   - How do you think he interprets his performance of school activities?
   - How do you think Dru anticipates his future engagement in school activities and how does this impact the choices he makes in the role of student?

3. Using MOHO concepts, explain the impact Dru's mother and grandmother have on his occupational participation.

HABITUATION

Habituation is an internalized readiness to demonstrate consistent patterns of behavior (Kielhofner, 2007). This readiness is supported by a person's habits and roles.

Children and their families participate in these habits and roles in recurring and stable ways according to the time of day, week, and year and the characteristics of the environment. Habits and roles help to organize our lives, thereby organizing our actions and encouraging successful participation.

When children respond to familiar situations in consistent ways, they are demonstrating a *habit*, or an acquired tendency to respond automatically to a specific circumstance or environment. Habits help children to be efficient and effective. For example, a child who has an organized routine when entering his or her classroom (hang up my backpack, then get out my homework folder and place it in my desk) will be able to quickly put his or her belongings into the proper place and prepare for the school day. Conversely, a child without a clear routine upon entering his or her classroom is required to process through each expectation each day and may not successfully complete the task of preparing for a new school day. Children and their families have habits of performance (the order in which clothes are put on), habits of routine (coming home from school and having a snack before starting homework), and habits of style (talkative and outgoing, or introspective and observant).

When a child identifies as a son or daughter, brother or sister, student, soccer player, band member, or worker, he or she is internalizing a *role*. Roles are culturally and socially defined, and are accompanied by a set of related actions and attitudes. For example, the role of a student is associated with the expectations of attending school, listening to the teacher, participating in activities, playing with classmates, and demonstrating learning on tests. Roles also help children and families define their relationships and actions with others; a child is expected to act differently when interacting with his or her teacher, mother, and best friend. A child who does not identify with any roles will have difficulty relating to others and interacting in socially and culturally valued activities.

Roles and habits have an organizing effect on a child and family's life over time. Routines and roles are traditionally different on the weekend (mow the lawn, organize a family picnic, or attend a religious service) compared to weekday roles and routines (daily chores, attend doctor's appointments, go to school). Routines and roles also shift according to the time of year (holiday celebrations, spring cleaning) and across the lifespan—while children are expected to play, as they grow older their role demands shift to being a student to eventually being a worker.

Learning Activity C

Identify and define the MOHO concepts and subconcepts that describe children's patterns of behavior.

Case Study #2: Habituation

By Stephanie McCammon, MS, OTR/L

Kelly is a 14-year-old African American young lady who was hospitalized in an adolescent psychiatric unit for aggression and self-harm behaviors. Kelly is part of the child welfare system and her guardian is the state. Due to her history of aggression and mental illness, she lives in a community facility designed to treat and care for adolescents with psychosocial difficulties. The facility placement staff plays the role of parent and supports Kelly in learning the skills needed to be successful in her life.

Kelly enjoys writing poetry, singing, journaling, and listening to music. She demonstrates poor social skills, limited process skills, low self-efficacy, and a decreased ability to manage her internal states. These difficulties limit her ability to successfully engage in her daily routine in her community placement and on the psychiatric unit. On the unit, Kelly tends to be more passive but benefits from verbal encouragement from staff to bolster belief in herself and her abilities. Kelly perceives herself as being a caring, kind person and takes pride in helping others. However, her ability to successfully fulfill the role of friend and group member within her context of a nontraditional family environment has been problematic.

As part of the psychiatric treatment team, the occupational therapist provides clinical assessment of occupational performance through structured activity, using MOHO as a guiding model. The occupational therapist collaborates with other disciplines and the client to create meaningful interventions to support participation in occupation both on the ward and in the client's community placement. As Kelly's hospitalization progressed, the treatment team felt it was important to address her limited ability to recognize positive experiences that occur throughout her day. Kelly's inability to express enjoyment or reflect upon her daily successes was not only impacting her sense of volition, but also limiting her ability to interact with others and manage her daily personal routines. Kelly's low sense of efficacy would cause her withdraw, interfering with her ability to meet role expectations.

At Kelly's weekly clinical staffing, the occupational therapist offered to help create a behavioral modification plan that used visual cues and rewards for meeting daily expectations. Other team members offered similar ideas to help Kelly reinforce her positive choices and attitude. Kelly was present for the last part of her staffing, however, and when asked to choose a reward she stated that she was "not a baby" and did not need rewards for her positive behaviors. She was highly resistant to the idea of "reward," and felt it was infantile.

After this meeting, the occupational therapist worked directly with Kelly and her primary nurse on the unit to identify strategies that would sustain more positive behaviors and help Kelly support herself in the completion of her daily routines. The occupational therapist suggested that the intervention incorporate her interest in writing so that it would have some intrinsic value to her. Kelly was very interested in a writing-based strategy and became invested in an activity that could further produce some original writing. It was decided that each day Kelly would write on a strip of paper positive things that she had done that day, and the pieces would be joined to form a paper chain link. At the end of a week, Kelly would be able to create a poem or creative writing using the positive thoughts from the chain links. The links allowed Kelly to visually recognize how many positive things she had accomplished, thereby supporting herself in the completion of everyday activities. She chose the color of construction paper for her chain links and was given all the necessary materials to complete a link every day. The chain was hung in Kelly's room on the unit.

Kelly remained invested in this intervention. Kelly felt the chain was a fun activity and she could generate a positive statement about herself with support from staff. She worked with a variety of staff to compose her statements every shift. Her comments included: "I was respectful to staff" and "I combed my hair pretty today." Kelly still needed a high level of support to help her organize and create a writing plan, but she was very motivated to engage in the production of something meaningful. Her behavior on the unit did improve over the course of her placement as she became more likely to recall positive choices even when she had a "bad day." Kelly would use past positive statements to get herself "back on track" for the next day, encouraging herself to participate in the unit activities and interact with other youth on the unit.

Interventions on this psychiatric unit seek to support the development of skills youths need to be effective, efficient, and safe community members and housemates. In Kelly's case, the intervention focused on increasing her self-efficacy and her ability to act as a member of her "home" environment and participate in its routines. Although this particular strategy was initiated in the hospital, the activity was shared with Kelly's placement staff to ensure that her development would continue once she returned to her home placement.

Nontraditional family environments, such as the one Kelly is a member of, have their own unique role demands and routines. Through ongoing communication between Kelly and her caregivers, the occupational therapist was able to help Kelly identify and use strategies that enabled her to meet the expectations of her home environment.

Case Study #2 Learning Activity

1. What are some of the roles Kelly identified that she had?
2. What factors interfere with Kelly's ability to meet role demands and engage in routines on the hospital ward and in her community placement?
3. What was the purpose of the intervention?
4. What MOHO concepts did this intervention use and attempt to address?

PERFORMANCE CAPACITY

A child's ability to participate in occupations is supported by the status of his or her physical and mental components as well as his or her subjective experience of living within his or her body. Occupational therapists use other frames of reference to measure, classify, and describe the status of physical and mental components of a child in order to explain problems of function that lead to limitations in participation. Therefore, MOHO acknowledges the importance of a child's physical and mental components but relies on a therapist's utilization of other frames of reference (e.g., Biomechanical, SI) to evaluate and explain those components. However, MOHO also recognizes that the subjective experience of living in a body influences how children perform and interact with their world. For example, a child with SI difficulties and gravitational insecurity may describe the experience of going down a slide as "falling into a black hole." This subjective experience, referred to as the *lived body experience*, influences a child's future occupational participation as well as his or her understanding of his or her body and world. A child's lived body experience influences his or her sense of capacity as much as the status of his or her physical and mental components. Awareness of a child's lived body experience requires an occupational therapist to consider the way a child experiences the world, which in turn helps the therapist recognize that addressing physical and mental components alone is not enough to transform a child's capacity to engage in occupations. The phenomological concept of the lived body is further explained in the text *The Model of Human Occupation: Theory and Application* (Kielhofner, 2007).

Learning Activity D

Identify and define the two aspects of performance capacity that impact children's ability to do occupations.

ENVIRONMENT

Whether with family or friends, at home or in school, or in a city or rural town, children and their families are impacted by their surroundings and their culture. All aspects of the environment, including man-made and natural spaces, objects, other community members, and local customs, offer either an opportunity or a barrier to participation in meaningful and culturally relevant occupations. Systematically recognizing environmental supports and constraints enables the occupational therapist to work in a more holistic manner and facilitate participation.

Every environment offers a combination of opportunities, resources, demands, and constraints (Kielhofner, 2007). A playground or tumble gym provides young children with the opportunity to explore, use their bodies, and experiment with vestibular and proprioceptive sensations. However, this same playground constrains the play of a child who uses a wheelchair for mobility if it is accessible only through steps. A teacher who provides verbal praise after a child completes half of his or her classwork is providing a resource that supports task completion within the corresponding environmental demand of on-task behavior. Family routines that support a smooth transition out of the house each morning before school enable a child to arrive on time each day, yet that same routine may not allow time for the child to actively participate in getting dressed or cleaning up after breakfast. A child who lives in a family with a steady income, transportation, and health insurance has different resources and opportunities than a child whose family does not have access to these resources due to chronic health conditions, problems in the local economy, or lack of social services. The environment impacts each person in a unique way depending on the qualities of the environment and the personal characteristics of each child, such as their sense of efficacy or capacity for performance.

MOHO describes the environment as consisting of physical elements and social elements (Kielhofner, 2007). The physical environment includes spaces and objects. Spaces can be both built and natural, and different spaces are associated with different demands and opportunities. A movie theater requires that a person sit still and remain relatively quiet until the movie is over; while a beach provides a choice of swimming, relaxing while enjoying the view, or playing in the sand. Objects are things that people interact with or use while engaging in a variety of activities. Whether a child chooses to play alone or with others may depend on the type of toys he or she has. For example, a mini-keyboard encourages solitary play while a box of dress-up clothes encourages imaginative play with others. Objects can also support children's engagement in occupations. For example, students regularly use pencils and paper, but may benefit from an alternative, such as using a computer to complete class assignments. Finally, objects are often associated with roles and interests. For example, a child learning to play baseball may never leave home without a catching glove, while a teenager's car is a sign of his or her growing independence and maturity.

Social groups and occupational forms/tasks make up the social aspect of the environment. Social groups are collections of people who come together for formal and informal purposes (Kielhofner, 2007). Social groups, which range from organized youth organizations to youth congregating at a local hang-out, also influence the actions and activities of the members. For example, a young child may yell, laugh, and play tag while playing with friends, while an adolescent student in a study group with peers may discuss homework problems, help a friend with spelling, and bring snacks to share with the group during breaks. As children grow older, the number of social groups they come into contact with increases and the types of social groups they engage in change; toddlers may be limited to social groups that involve their family, but as children begin to attend school and become more involved in the community they become increasingly involved in different social groups that include peers and adults. In this way, social groups impact a child's roles and related role behavior. Like other environmental factors, social groups can either encourage participation (e.g., a sports team that includes children with disabilities and without disabilities) or restrict involvement (e.g., a school that is hesitant to place a child in an inclusion class).

Another aspect of the social environment is the presence of occupational forms/tasks, or conventionalized ways of doing things. Occupational forms/tasks include the actions and manners that characterize a certain activity and are connected to the meaning of the activity. This includes activities referred to previously such as playing a game of baseball, being in a study group, or taking notes in class. Occupational forms/tasks are shaped by culture and can be established by law, such as an Individualized Education Program (IEP) meeting. Occupational forms/tasks can also be influenced by local customs, such as sitting on the front porch after supper. Occupational forms/tasks have varying levels of formality, expectations, and flexibility. The opportunity a child has to participate in culturally valued forms is often determined by the flexibility of that form, such as the previous example of a sports team incorporating wheelchairs into the team play.

Learning Activity E

1. Identify the four things that every environment offers. Identify and define the aspects that make up children's environments.
2. Define and explain the idea of environmental impact.

Case Study #3: Environment

By Staci Ollar, OTR/L

Evan is a 4-year, 3-month-old girl who was adopted from an orphanage in Moldova when she was 18 months old. Evan was previously given a medical diagnosis of "motor dyspraxia," and she received private occupational therapy at a rehabilitation center on a weekly basis. While enrolled in preschool, her mother requested a school-based occupational therapy evaluation due to apparent fine motor and sensory delays. Both of Evan's parents are teachers within the school district she attends and are aware of the resources available to Evan within the school district. During the evaluation, her mother described the orphanage as understaffed with an apparent sensory deprived environment. Evan also has a younger sister and older brother. Her mother describes her as a loving child who doesn't realize her own strength or recognize personal space. This affects her relationship with her siblings and peers, as Evan often plays alone or with adults. Her mother was tearful when expressing her fears of Evan's peer relationships or lack thereof. Evan's preschool teacher describes her as having a low frustration tolerance during prewriting and seated activities.

The therapist assessed Evan using the Peabody Developmental Motor Scales (Folio & Fewell, 2000), the Beery VMI (Beery, Buktenica, & Beery, 2004), and the Pediatric Volitional Questionnaire (Basu, Kafkes, Geist, & Kielhofner, 2002).

Evan's parents and teacher also completed a sensory questionnaire. The PVQ was completed during a seated classroom activity and during free play on the playground in order to identify possible volitional difficulties and activities Evan enjoyed and felt more competent doing. She demonstrated great difficulty sitting and attending for longer than 2 minutes during the Peabody, VMI, and class activity, and on the playground she spent the majority of her time spinning on a tire swing. The PVQ environmental form (see Figure 4-7 later in this chapter) was used to examine the differences in the two environments and identify the environmental aspects that supported Evan's participation. Assessment results revealed delayed fine motor, visual motor, and self-help skills. Upper extremity strength, range of motion, cutting, and perceptual skills (constructional) were within normal limits. The sensory screening revealed modulation dysfunction.

As Evan was demonstrating fine motor and perceptual difficulties in some areas and not in others, the occupational therapist decided to use environmental strategies, modifications, and/or adaptations that would encourage Evan's participation in a variety of school activities and take advantage of her abilities. The therapist wanted to focus on making changes to the environment that would provide Evan with things she enjoyed and support her in feeling effective and competent when performing activities. In addition, these strategies would also address Evan's sensory needs. The therapist consulted with Evan's preschool teacher to describe Evan's sensory needs and to identify strategies that would support Evan's success in the classroom. The occupational therapist suggested a sensory-based writing program, and she and the teacher identified a program that Evan could benefit from. A list of proprioceptive activities was generated so that the teacher could ask Evan to be a class helper while simultaneously providing her with sensory input that would prepare her for seated activities. The list included things like stacking chairs, pushing the supply cart, wiping the chalkboard clean, and carrying books. The therapist also provided Evan with objects that would provide sensory input and improve her attention and classroom performance. This included a seat cushion, a weighted vest, fidget toys like putty and stress balls, and headphones to reduce classroom noise. In addition, Evan's new handwriting program included manipulatives such as shapes, chalk, a wet sponge, and a personal writing slate.

The therapist also asked Evan's mother if they would like to implement sensory strategies at home. The parents were interested in trying the strategies to see if they supported Evan and her participation at home and in the community without greatly impacting her other siblings. The therapist taught the Wilbarger protocol (Wilbarger & Wilbarger, 1991) to the parents and supported them in identifying times to implement the program within their current routine. In addition, the therapist explained the impact heavy work and proprioceptive input can have on attention and regulation and suggested strategies such as bear hugs in the morning, carrying grocery bags into the house, bringing in firewood, shoveling snow (as appropriate for her age), carrying laundry baskets upstairs, and using a lightly inflated camp cushion in church.

Evan's teacher and parents reported more on-task behavior in class and during other quiet activities such as church. In addition, Evan was proud of being a good helper for her teacher, and felt she did a good job performing her helper role. Evan's sensory objects and strategies improved her attention and ability to manage frustration, which enabled her to focus on practicing writing and other fine motor skills such as zipping her jacket. Evan's classmates also took an interest in her sensory toys, creating an opportunity for Evan to interact with her peers in a positive way. However, Evan was sometimes reluctant to share and needed support to avoid becoming upset. Since all the children were interested and motivated by Evan's objects, the teacher and the therapist decided to provide all students with fidget toys and the handwriting program manipulatives at their desks. In addition, a sensory corner with several therapy balls, a weighted blanket, a body sock, and a listening station (with headphones) was created and available to all students during "center" free playtime. Within this comfortable environment, Evan began to interact and play with some of her peers. Noticing this success, Evan's mother asked the therapist to identify similar strategies that could encourage interaction between Evan and her siblings and peers in her community.

Difficulties with sensory modulation greatly affect how a student learns and feels about his or her ability to be effective and competent. MOHO can help illuminate how the environment impacts a student's performance and contributes to his or her sense of personal causation. The occupational therapist plays a crucial role in educating parents, teachers, and administrative staff and implementing environmental strategies to improve a student's classroom and community performance. In Evan's case, her parents were invited to a sensory seminar and introduced to another parent in the school district who also adopted a child from Moldova with sensory disturbances. Coincidentally, the parents soon discovered their children were adopted from the same orphanage and were able to provide support to each other and share successful strategies that facilitated their children's participation at school, at home, and in their community.

Case Study #3 Learning Activity

1. List the environments that were considered in this case study. What were the physical and social aspects of each of these environments/settings?

2. Before the occupational therapist became involved, what environmental demands and constraints were impacting Evan's participation in occupations?

3. What modifications did the occupational therapist make to provide Evan with resources and opportunities that encouraged participation? (For example, how did the occupational therapist modify the occupational form/task of handwriting instruction in the classroom?)

Summary

This section discussed the main concepts of MOHO, including the personal characteristics of volition, habituation, and performance capacity. The physical and social aspects of the environment were also reviewed along with the impact an environment has on an individual depending on the opportunities, resources, demands, or constraints presented in the environment.

Next, this chapter will review the different ways that people interact with and participate in their world.

— Section II —

Dimensions of Doing

In daily life, participation in occupations falls along a continuum of "doing." When considering a day at school, children engage in roles as students, complete class assignments, and process information and utilize motor actions to engage in those activities. We can analyze this continuum of doing at the levels of participation, performance, and skill.

As MOHO is a top-down model, the discussion of the levels of doing will begin with occupational participation and continue along the continuum to skill.

Occupational Participation

Consistent with the World Health Organization (2001) and the *Practice Framework* (AOTA, 2002), occupational participation refers to a person's involvement in life situations through engagement in work, play, or activities of daily living that are part of the social and cultural context and necessary for well-being (Kielhofner, 2007). Influenced by individual characteristics and the environment, occupational participation is both personal and contextual. In western society, children are expected to participate in self-care activities (such as getting dressed, eating meals, picking up after themselves), attend school, and interact with family and friends. The nature of a child's capacities, interests, values, and environmental opportunities may determine what free time activities will be chosen at school (e.g., music corner or sand table) and in the community (e.g., video games or neighborhood playground). Whether a child is participating as a student, family member, or member of a sports team, this participation is associated with a related cluster of activities and occupations. For example, when participating as a student, a child may be required to take notes in class and answer questions, while a child participating on a soccer team is expected to attend practice in order to learn how to move a soccer ball down the field. Doing these related activities demonstrates occupational performance, the next level of doing.

OCCUPATIONAL PERFORMANCE

When children engage in goal-directed activities, they are performing, or going through the demonstration of an occupational form/task. Occupational performance refers to "doing" of occupational forms/tasks. A student writing and taking notes in the classroom is performing an occupation. Occupational performance is influenced by roles (being a student is associated with the performance of note taking) and habits (the patterns of actions a student uses while taking notes). Additionally, the environment impacts a person's occupational performance, as the environment can provide resources and opportunities that facilitate performance or demands and constraints that restrict performance. Using our example of taking notes, if a student has difficulty writing with a pencil (a combination of skills), an environment that provides alternative ways of doing the form of note-taking (e.g., a keyboard, pencil grips, slant board, or typed handouts) continues to support occupational performance.

OCCUPATIONAL SKILL

When participating in activities, children demonstrate certain actions associated with that occupational form/task. For example, when learning to use the commode, children must process the sensation to void, communicate their need to use the restroom, and use a series of fine and gross motor actions to remove their clothing and sit on the commode seat. These observable, goal-directed actions that emerge from the person's engagement with his or her environment during an occupation are skills (Kielhofner, 2007). Unlike performance capacity, which is an individual's underlying ability, skills emerge in the process of doing an occupation and are reflective of a person's volition, habituation, performance capacity, and the impact of the environment.

MOHO identifies three main sets of skills: motor skills, process skills, and communication and interaction skills.

Motor skills refer to moving self or objects related to the task (Fisher, 1999). This includes actions such as bending, manipulating, lifting, and moving objects from one place to another. *Process skills* are demonstrated when actions are logically sequenced, tools and materials are used appropriately, and performance is adapted when problems are encountered (Fisher, 1999). *Communication and interaction skills* convey intentions and needs with others in order to act together and include gesturing, physical contact, speaking, and being assertive (Forsyth & Kielhofner, 1999). Tools that can be used to assess children's skills will be discussed later in this chapter.

Handwriting requires a variety of motor and process skills such as attending, sequencing actions, grasping, and stabilizing the body. These skills we observe are influenced by the nature of the writing object, the topic of the assignment, how quiet or distracting the classroom is, and the child's physical and mental capacities.

1. Identify and define the levels of doing, and describe the MOHO concepts that influence each level of doing.
2. Differentiate between the MOHO concepts of skill and performance capacity.
3. Discuss how a child's impairment could impact each of these levels of doing.

Case Study #4: Dimensions of Doing

By Susan A. Swidler, MOT, OTR/L, IMC

BACKGROUND

Sam is a 5-year-old boy with a diagnosis of right hemiplegic cerebral palsy. He was born at 37 weeks gestation, with some evidence of regulatory compromises including difficulty feeding early on due to an inability to stay alert/awake. Sam has been receiving direct occupational, physical, speech, and developmental therapy since he was 10 months of age. Current programming includes occupational therapy twice per week, physical therapy twice per week, and speech therapy one time per week. Sam wears a handsplint to facilitate thumb abduction and wrist extension of the right hand and a right foot orthotic. He has participated in forced use casting over the past year and a half. His left arm has been casted four times for a period of 1 month at a time to encourage active use of the right upper extremity, showing positive gains. During intervention, Sam receives electrical stimulation to his right wrist extensors and triceps during active reaching in functional activities as well as to his abdominal and paraspinal muscles to aid in activation of the trunk musculature. Sam participates in electrical stimulation in the home environment three times per week to his paraspinal muscles. He will be starting kindergarten in the fall.

ASSESSING OCCUPATIONAL PARTICIPATION

The Short Child Occupational Profile (SCOPE) was recently administered to Sam as a way to identify strengths and occupational difficulties and to monitor progress in occupational participation. Most assessments previously used for testing purposes have presented Sam as having multiple deficits and do not tend to convey his sense of volition and positive attitude, nor account for the support provided by his family. The SCOPE was chosen as a tool that might better reflect Sam and his family's strengths, as well as identify areas of need. The SCOPE was used in combination with motor assessments, creating a more holistic evaluation of Sam's current situation. The occupational therapist completed the SCOPE based on current knowledge of Sam and also sought feedback from the rest of the therapy team when rating the SCOPE. Direct observation and clinical judgment were also utilized for administration of the tool. Sam's mother attends therapy sessions and close communication and collaboration with the family allowed for the therapist to answer questions regarding Sam's functioning outside of the clinic environment.

On the SCOPE (Figure 4-2), Sam scored strongest in the areas of volition, habituation, and communication and interaction skills. In all three areas, he received three "Fair" (F) ratings and one "Allows" (A) rating (see Figure 4-2 for the meaning of these ratings). Sam demonstrated strength in the area of volition. Sam is able to identify activities that are enjoyable and satisfying to him and expresses his enjoyment during engagement.

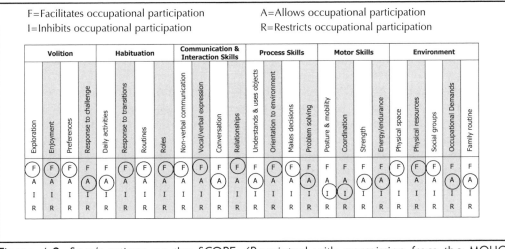

Figure 4-2. Sam's ratings on the SCOPE. (Reprinted with permission from the MOHO Clearinghouse, Dept. of Occupational Therapy, University of Illinois at Chicago.)

Habituation items also facilitate Sam's occupational participation—he is aware of his roles, routines, and habits. Sam's roles include being a son, a brother, a friend, a player, and a student.

Sam's mother had the following comments based on the areas addressed by the SCOPE:

"Sam loves to run, climb, crash, and explore his environment. He is fearless, and sometimes needs supervision to pay attention to safety. He easily expresses enjoyment, but is equally as quick to express frustration when tasks are hard. Sam is very verbal and knows what he likes. Sam is willing to attempt new and challenging activities, although he is quick to ask for assistance, especially with tasks requiring the use of both hands. Sam knows routines and is familiar with common daily chores and self-care tasks. He requires assistance to put on his shoes, button his pants, zip his jacket, and needs help when using a knife. Transitions are easy for Sam. He has no problem following routines and can tell you the sequence of regular routines he participates in. Communication is an area of strength for Sam. He demonstrates good eye contact and really uses facial expressions to get his point across! He sometimes has difficulty coordinating breathing during an activity—he really has to work hard since he is not very strong and has a hard time working with his hands."

Sam's scores on the SCOPE indicated that his motor skills could be interfering with his occupational participation—he received two "Inhibits" (I) and two "Allows" (A). He demonstrates more challenges when performing discrete motor tasks due to his motor impairments, so the occupational therapist collaborated with the physical therapist to complete this section of the SCOPE. Together they determined that Sam has difficulty maintaining postural control during bilateral and fine motor activities. He demonstrates multiple compensations during gross and fine motor tasks, such as leaning against the table or working with his arms close to his side. Sam has difficulty with throwing and catching a ball, using scissors for cutting, writing, and manipulating fasteners. It is difficult for Sam to grade force and speed for gross and fine motor tasks. Because of these difficulties, Sam tires during meals and requires increased time to eat.

In the area of process skills, Sam received two "Facilitates" (F) and two "Allows" (A). Sam demonstrates appropriate imaginary play using different materials in his surroundings, and he is able to help with age-appropriate household chores. However, his physical limitations with his right hand often impair his ability to perform activities, especially those that involve the use of objects. Sam often requests help when physically challenged rather than modifying his actions or attempting to solve the problem on his own. When he is angry or frustrated because he is unable to solve a problem or meet a challenge, Sam has difficulty expressing himself. He will often repeat "No" over and over, and sometimes he will cry.

The environment proved to facilitate Sam's occupational participation. Overall, the environment provides Sam with opportunities and resources, but occasionally restricts his occupational performance. For example, Sam does not have a good chair in the home environment where his feet can be flat on the floor. This could be a problem as he enters kindergarten and begins to complete homework assignments. Sometimes, the family and babysitter tend to do too much for Sam in the home setting, when all he needs to participate in certain tasks is increased time, encouragement, and minimal assistance. However, often the family routine does not allow enough time for Sam to perform self-care tasks independently even when he has the skills.

GOALS AND INTERVENTION STRATEGIES

The SCOPE assisted in providing an occupation-based framework for the development of goals for intervention. Occupational therapy continues to be recommended twice a week to address Sam's hypotonic muscle tone, postural stability, and related positioning. However, based upon the results of the SCOPE, direct discussion with the family, and clinical observations, new treatment goals were developed for Sam and the therapist implemented corresponding intervention strategies she knew Sam enjoyed. For example, the therapist would use obstacle courses that included both gross and fine motor challenges, so he could have more opportunities to "run, climb, crash, and explore" in between the more difficult fine motor activities.

Treatment goals will shift from focusing primarily on Sam's postural and motor difficulties (such as the acquisition of improved motor skills for bilateral coordination, fine motor, and activities of daily living) to incorporate more family involvement to better assist Sam and his family. The therapist will facilitate the family's identification of strategies that will allow Sam to do things safely and independently at home, and work with Sam's parents so they may better match their demands and expectations to Sam's abilities. The therapist will especially focus on Sam's participation in valued role-related routines and activities, such as playing with his brother, getting dressed, and contributing to house chores. When Sam begins kindergarten in the fall, the occupational therapist will also work with Sam's teacher to identify resources and supports in the classroom environment that can be utilized to facilitate his participation.

Case Study #4 Learning Activity

1. Using the continuum of the levels of doing, consider Sam's occupational participation as a family member.
2. How does occupational performance differ when he is enacting the role of "brother" vs. doing self-care activities?
3. What skills are impacting performance in these two areas?
4. To support Sam's participation as a family member, how did the occupation therapist address Sam's performance and skills?

Table 4-1
LEVELS OF DOING

Levels of Doing	Examples			
Occupational Participation	Self-care	Being a student	Helping family with chores	Having friends
Occupational Performance	Brushing teeth, getting dressed	Taking notes, finishing homework	Setting the table, picking up toys	Sharing toys, playing imaginative games like "house"
Occupational Skills	Manipulating, sequencing, reaching	Sequencing, manipulating, reaching	Sequencing, walking, reaching, calibrating	Sequencing, speaking, manipulating

(Adapted from Kielhofner, G. [2007]. *The model of human occupation: Theory and application* [4th ed.]. Baltimore: Lippincott, Williams & Wilkins.)

SUMMARY

This section discussed the levels of doing: occupational participation, occupational performance, and skill. Refer to Table 4-1 for an example of different types of occupational participation that are common to children in western mainstream culture. Each of these dimensions is influenced by a child's characteristics (volition, habituation, and performance capacity), as well as the opportunities, resources, demands, and constraints of the environment. Over time, participating in a variety of occupations results in a sense of occupational competence and occupational identity, leading to occupational adaptation. These concepts will be discussed next.

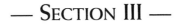

— SECTION III —

Demonstrating Occupational Adaptation

Occupational adaptation results when two interrelated elements, occupational competence and occupational identity, are constructed and maintained over time within the context of a person's environment (Kielhofner, 2007). Occupational identity is a composite sense of who one is currently (student, son or daughter, friend) and who one wishes to become in the future (girlfriend or boyfriend, worker). A person's imagined future as an occupational being is influenced by his or her past participation—a student who does not do well in school will not imagine him- or herself as a future college student.

The set of elements that contribute to one's occupational identity when experienced and accumulated over time include (Kielhofner, 2007):

- One's sense of capacity and effectiveness
- Activities that one finds interesting and enjoyable
- One's internalized roles and relationships and the associated obligations and values
- A life that includes a sense of familiar routines

Figure 4-3. The process of occupational adaptation. (Adapted from Kielhofner, G. [2007]. *The model of human occupation: Theory and application* [4th ed.]. Baltimore: Lippincott, Williams & Wilkins.)

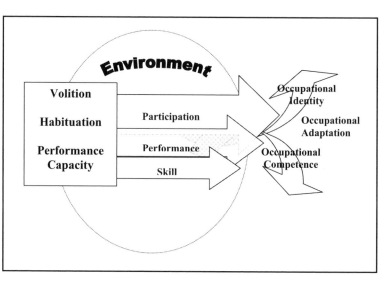

- Perceptions of the supportiveness or demands of the environment
- An experience of one's lived body

In short, occupational identity serves as both a means of self-definition and as a blueprint for upcoming action (Kielhofner, 2007).

Sustaining a pattern of participation that reflects one's occupational identity leads to a sense of occupational competence. Occupational competence is the result of acting out an occupational identity, which includes (Kielhofner, 2007):

- Meeting expectations and performance standards associated with roles and values
- Maintaining a routine and organizing life in a way that enables a person to meet responsibilities
- Participating in a range of occupations that are interesting, satisfying, and provide a sense of ability and control
- Following one's values and taking actions to meet values and goals

Children and their families develop a sense of occupational competence when family members can contribute to the family, meet society's role expectations (such as being a student or worker), and meet family goals such as owning a home or helping a child obtain his or her degree. Occupational therapists can provide resources and facilitate the skills that support children's occupational engagement in school, at home, and in their community in order to enable their sense of occupational competence.

In summary, personal characteristics such as volition, habituation, and performance capacity, in interaction with the environment during participation, lead to an occupational identify and sense of competence. This process of occupational adaptation is pictured in Figure 4-3.

Learning Activity G

1. Define occupational identity and describe how it impacts occupational adaptation.
2. Define occupational competence and describe how it impacts occupational adaptation.

Case Study #5: Occupational Adaptation in MOHO

By Susan M. Cahill, MAEA, OTR/L

Javion is an 8-year, 2-month-old boy with a medical diagnosis of autism. He is currently included in a second grade classroom with 23 other students. In addition to receiving special education resource services, he receives occupational therapy and speech and language therapy. Javion also benefits from assistance provided by a teacher's aide who is assigned to his classroom.

Javion communicates through words and pictures. He verbalizes sentences up to six words in length to state a command, preference, or immediate need. Javion lacks social and emotional reciprocity and has difficulty carrying on a conversation without the use of visual aids.

Javion enjoys reading and reads at grade level. He has an extensive sight word vocabulary, but does not generally respond to comprehension questions beyond the literal level. Javion consistently passes his weekly math tests and can complete subtraction problems that involve regrouping. His teacher reports that over the past 3 months it has become more and more challenging to get him to initiate academic tasks, as well as remain focused until the completion of an activity. She also reported that Javion no longer appears to be motivated by the classroom behavior management system, which includes opportunities to earn reinforcements such as stickers, "no homework" passes, and a positive phone call home.

Increased talking or noise within the classroom can cause Javion to get off track. Once Javion has reached his sensory threshold he will engage in behaviors such as hand flapping, rocking in his chair, quickly shaking his head from side to side, or squeezing his head. When Javion becomes frustrated or overstimulated, he is able to state that he wants/needs a break by saying "I need a break" or by asking for the specific sensory activity.

UNDERSTANDING JAVION'S PERSPECTIVE

The team determined that more information was needed regarding Javion's own perception of his school experience. Because of Javion's limited communication abilities, the team had made many assumptions about what was meaningful to him. In order to come up with reinforcements that were motivating to Javion, they decided to use the Child Occupational Self Assessment (COSA) to find out what he valued, as well as what he perceived as areas of personal strength in the classroom environment.

Prior to administering the COSA, the occupational therapist worked with the speech and language pathologist to assess Javion's understanding of the rating scale responses used in the assessment. Armed with a list of Javion's known likes and dislikes, the occupational therapist developed a grid similar to the one on the COSA reporting form and substituted COSA items for the ones on Javion's list. In addition, she numbered the items and highlighted the responses related to Competence in blue and the responses related to Values in yellow. She then developed a checklist similar to the ones used by Javion during classroom instruction so that he would be sure to choose a "blue" answer and a "yellow" answer for each item.

Once it had been determined that Javion understood the rating scale used on the COSA, the therapist prepared to administer it. She again numbered the items and highlighted the responses accordingly to keep with the routine that had been established. The occupational therapist and Javion read the directions and the items on the checklist out loud together. Javion completed the COSA in approximately 15 minutes stopping only once to comment on a train that he thought he heard outside.

Once Javion finished the COSA he asked to lie under the beanbag chair and take a break. The occupational therapist agreed with this request. In the meantime, she reviewed his responses on the COSA and circled the items that he indicated "I have a big problem doing this" (Figure 4-4).

Javion reported having a "big problem" with the following items: having enough time to do what he likes, keeping his mind on what he is doing, finishing classwork on time, asking the teacher questions, and continuing to work when it gets hard. Javion also specified that these items held a great deal of value to him, as he rated them all either "really important to me" or "most important to me."

Once Javion had returned from his break, he and his occupational therapist reviewed the answers he had chosen for each item on the COSA. The occupational therapist encouraged Javion to elaborate on the items listed above. During their conversation, the therapist learned that Javion felt sad when his teacher was not smiling. He recognized that his teacher was not pleased with the recent change in his behavior. In addition, he expressed that he did not like it when students that sat at his table got up to sharpen their pencils during independent work time. It was also difficult for him to work when his classmates were talking. Javion indicated that he often did not ask for help because the classroom rule was to work independently.

Javion and therapist also reviewed the items that he endorsed as being "good at." Javion reported that he was good at doing things with his classmates and his friends, but that this was not really important to him. He also indicated that he was "good at" getting his homework done, taking care of his things, and choosing what he wants to do.

The therapist discussed with Javion some of the concerns adults had about his class performance using terms that he understood. Now knowing what Javion valued and which areas he felt competent in, she helped him to develop a list of positive reinforcers or "things to work for" throughout the day.

Javion felt competent completing homework assignments and saw value in doing so, yet he struggled with completing class assignments. Javion's occupational therapist and teacher devised a system where he would get three passes per day to take home three class assignments of his choice. Stickers did not motivate Javion to initiate a task or remain focused, but through the interview process he reported that he liked to see his teacher smile. The occupational therapist modified Javion's behavior chart so that instead of receiving stickers, he would receive mini color-copied photos of his teacher. Additionally, Javion did not ask the teacher for help when he needed. The teacher agreed to hold up a cue card to the class when she was presenting more complicated material. This would be a visual cue to Javion, as well as to the rest of the class, that it was an appropriate time to ask questions.

Javion's environment also had to be modified in order to support his performance in the classroom. The team knew that Javion was sensitive to sounds, which is why he was seated furthest away from the pencil sharpener. However, the team had not recognized that one of the students who sat at Javion's table was getting up two to three times during each independent work time to sharpen his pencil, get a drink, or throw something in the garbage can. Changing this student's seat would eliminate some of the distractions that Javion was being challenged with on a daily basis. In addition, the classroom teacher set up an office area in a quiet corner of the room that was blocked off by a partition so that Javion could retreat if he was becoming too distracted by his classmates' talking.

The COSA assisted the team in learning more about Javion's perceptions regarding his own sense of occupational competence, as well as the value he placed on daily occupations. It provided Javion with a voice and an opportunity to direct his services. In addition, it afforded the team with a platform on which to begin addressing Javion's current needs in the classroom.

Myself	I have a big problem doing this	I have a little problem doing this	I do this OK	I am really good at doing this	Not really important to me	Important to me	Really important to me	Most important of all to me
Keep my body clean			X				X	
Dress myself			X				X	
Eat my meals without any help			X				X	
Buy something myself		X					X	
Get my chores done			X				X	
Get enough sleep			X				X	
Have enough time to do things I like	X							X
Take care of my things				X				X
Get around from one place to another			X				X	
Choose things that I want to do				X			X	
Keep my mind on what I am doing	X							X
Do things with my family			X				X	
Do things with my friends				X		X		
Do things with my classmates				X		X		
Follow classroom rules			X				X	
Finish my work in class on time	X							X
Get my homework done				X				X
Ask my teacher questions when I need to	X						X	
Make others understand my ideas			X				X	
Think of ways to do things when I have a problem			X				X	
Keep working on something even when it gets hard	X						X	
Calm myself down when I am upset		X					X	
Make my body do what I want it to do			X			X		
Use my hands to work with things			X				X	
Finish what I am doing without getting tired too soon			X			X		

Figure 4-4. Javion's responses on the COSA. (Reprinted with permission from the MOHO Clearinghouse, Dept. of Occupational Therapy, University of Illinois at Chicago.)

Case Study #5 Learning Activity

1. Using Javion's responses, what things are contributing to his sense of occupational identity as a student (including his values, sense of capacity, and internalized roles)?

2. Using Javion's responses, what things are contributing to his sense of occupational competence as a student (including his ability to meet expectations, participate in valued roles, and organize his routine)?

— SECTION IV —

Clinical Reasoning Using the Model of Human Occupation

When using a theory in practice, therapists must understand how to incorporate the tenants of the theory into their therapeutic reasoning process. Therapeutic reasoning, a client-focused reasoning process (Kielhofner, 2007), requires the therapist to consider the unique circumstances of the client and the concepts of the model simultaneously. This sophisticated process can be broken down into the following phases (Kielhofner, 2007):

*   Generate questions to guide data collection
*   Collect information about the person's occupational life
*   Develop an explanation of the client's circumstances based on his or her information and theory
*   Develop decisions for actions with the client and implement therapeutic goals and strategies

These phases are not sequential, but are addressed throughout the occupational therapy process. Although the therapist may spend the most time generating questions and collecting information during evaluation, during the course of intervention as new insights are gained, the therapist should use this information to reassess his or her explanation of the client's circumstances and adjust goals and strategies accordingly. The therapeutic reasoning process is both client-centered and theoretically driven as each of these phases is influenced by the client's individual characteristics and the therapist's knowledge of MOHO (Kielhofner, 2007). A detailed explanation of the therapeutic reasoning process is covered in Kielhofner (2007), but this section will review the MOHO-based questions that can be used to guide data collection and develop an explanation of the client and his or her family's circumstances in pediatric practice.

USING QUESTIONS TO SUPPORT THERAPEUTIC REASONING WITH THE MODEL OF HUMAN OCCUPATION

A therapist begins to work with a child or adolescent and his or her family and wants to understand what factors are impacting the client's occupational participation. How can therapists begin to tease out the various issues contributing to the client's occupational adaptation? The first step is to ask broad questions about that child, his or her family, and his or her circumstances that are based on MOHO concepts. The therapist should begin by asking questions that address occupational adaptation and participation, and then move on to ask questions related to the client's characteristics and the impact of the environment. By beginning the therapeutic reasoning process with questions that are occupation- and theory-based, the therapist naturally continues this occupational focus during assessment, explanation, and goal setting. In this way, these general questions support an occupation-centered therapy process.

Table 4-2 provides general questions generated from the main concepts of MOHO theory. These questions should then drive further data collection through informal interview, observation, and formalized assessment procedures. The answers to these questions, obtained during data collection, begin to illuminate the areas of strength and the factors that may be interfering with occupational participation and successful adaptation. When a therapist identifies a particular area that is causing a client to have difficulties in his or her occupational engagement, the therapist may need to ask more specific questions. For a detailed accounting of these specific questions, therapists should refer to Kielhofner (2007).

Learning Activity H

1. Identify the phases of therapeutic reasoning.
2. Describe how asking theory-based questions supports the implementation of theory in practice.
3. Using one of the case studies in this chapter, demonstrate how MOHO questions can be used to identify personal and environmental factors requiring further assessment.
4. Discuss how the MOHO process of clinical reasoning is aligned with the AOTA's *Occupational Therapy Practice Framework*.

— SECTION V —

Technology for Practice (Assessments, Protocols, and Resources)

Using a model in practice requires that technologies for application are available, such as assessment tools, treatment protocols, and other resources that demonstrate the use of the model in practice such as case studies (Kielhofner, 2004). Whether assessments use standardized or naturalistic data collection methods, theoretically based assessments allow a therapist to gather and analyze information according to the propositions of the model in keeping with the process of therapeutic reasoning. Resources such as intervention protocols support the development of intervention strategies that are aligned with the concepts of the model. Case studies illuminate the process of clinical reasoning with the model and can be used to demonstrate the application of the model with an individual client or in an intervention program. MOHO provides such technology for application in order to bridge the gap between theory and practice.

Table 4-2

GENERAL QUESTIONS TO SUPPORT MOHO THERAPEUTIC REASONING WITH CHILDREN AND THEIR FAMILIES

MOHO Concept	Corresponding Questions
Occupational Identity	What is the child's sense of who he or she has been, is, and wishes to become? What is the family's sense of who this child has been or is, and what do they wish him or her to become? How do family members view themselves as occupational beings in relation to this child in the past, present, and future (e.g., parent, sibling)?
Occupational Competence	To what extent has this child sustained a pattern of occupational participation over time that reflects his or her occupational identity? To what extent have important people in this child's life sustained patterns of occupational participation over time that reflect their occupational identity in relation to this child (e.g., caregiving, playmate)?
Participation	Does the child currently engage in work, play, and ADL that are part of his or her sociocultural context and that are desired and/or necessary for his or her well-being? What work, play, and ADL activities does the family consider to be desired and/or necessary for the well-being of their child?
Performance	Can this child do the occupational forms/tasks that are part of the work, play, and ADL activities that make up, or should make up, his or her life? What occupational forms/tasks does the family expect the child to do as part of his or her work, play, and ADL activities? Can the family do the occupational forms/tasks that support their participation in occupations related to this child (e.g., changing a diaper, helping with homework)?
Skill	Does the child exhibit the necessary communication/interaction, motor, and process skills to perform what he or she needs and wants to do? Does the family support the child in developing the necessary communication/interaction, motor, and process skills needed for his or her participation and development?
Environment	What impact do the opportunities, resources, constraints, and demands (or lack of demands) of the environment have on how this child thinks, feels, and acts? What impact do the opportunities, resources, constraints, and demands of the environment have on how this family thinks, feels, and acts? How do the opportunities, resources, constraints, or demands provided by spaces, objects, occupational forms/tasks, and social groups affect the child's skill, performance, and participation?

continued

Table 4-2 (continued) GENERAL QUESTIONS TO SUPPORT MOHO THERAPEUTIC REASONING WITH CHILDREN AND THEIR FAMILIES	
MOHO Concept	*Corresponding Questions*
Volition	What is this child's view of his or her personal capacity and effectiveness, and how does it affect the choice, experience, interpretation, and anticipation of doing things? What convictions and sense of obligations does this child have and how does it affect the choice, experience, interpretation, and anticipation of doing things? What are this child's interests and how do they affect the choice, experience, interpretation, and anticipation of doing things?
Habituation	What are this child's habits and how do they influence the patterns of what he or she routinely does? What are the roles with which this child identifies with and how do they influence what he or she routinely does?
Performance Capacity	What objective and subjective factors influence this child's performance capacity?

(Adapted from Kielhofner, G. [2007]. *The model of human occupation: Theory and application* [4th ed.]. Baltimore: Lippincott, Williams & Wilkins.)

Several assessments based on MOHO have been developed for use with children and youth. The development of these assessments represents a collaborative effort between clinicians and researchers who engaged in a "scholarship of practice" (Hammel, Finlayson, Kielhofner, Helfrich, & Peterson, 2002; Kielhofner, 2005). The result is the creation of assessments that are clinically relevant, theoretically based, and psychometrically sound. Assessments for children and youth address a range of MOHO concepts, including volition, habituation, environment, skills, competence, and performance and participation. A short description of each MOHO assessment that has been developed for use with children and youth follows, but therapists interested in learning more about the assessments should refer to the text *The Model of Human Occupation: Theory and Application* (Kielhofner, 2007) or the assessment manuals. Case studies within this chapter also illustrate the use of some of these tools in practice.

THE CHILD OCCUPATIONAL SELF ASSESSMENT

The COSA (Keller, Kafkes, Basu, Federico, & Kielhofner, 2005) is a pediatric self-assessment that provides young clients with an opportunity to provide input into the evaluation and intervention planning process. The COSA has 25 items that cover a range of everyday activities, including self-care ("keep my body clean"), school tasks ("finish my work in class on time"), social activities ("do things with my family"), and family-related activities ("get my chores done"). For each item, clients reflect on how competent they feel doing each activity, and how important each activity is to them. The child's perception of competence when participating in the activities on the COSA reveals their sense of occupational competence, while their reported level of importance relates to the child's values

Myself	I have a big problem doing this	I have a little problem doing this	I do this ok	I am really good at doing this	Not really important to me	Important to me	Really important to me	Most important of all to me
Keep working on something even when it gets hard	☹ ☹	☹	☺	☺ ☺	★	★ ★	★ ★ ★	★ ★ ★ ★
Calm myself down when I get upset	☹ ☹	☹	☺	☺ ☺	★	★ ★	★ ★ ★	★ ★ ★ ★
Make my body do what I want it to do	☹ ☹	☹	☺	☺ ☺	★	★ ★	★ ★ ★	★ ★ ★ ★

Figure 4-5. Excerpt from the COSA rating form. (Reprinted with permission from the MOHO Clearinghouse, Dept. of Occupational Therapy, University of Illinois at Chicago.)

and can facilitate a better understanding of their occupational identity. Asking children to provide input to the evaluation and intervention process supports a collaborative and client-centered occupational therapy process.

Targeted to children ages 8 to 12, the COSA has also been used successfully with youth up to age 17 (Keller, Kafkes, & Kielhofner, 2005; Keller & Kielhofner, 2005). Visual cues (faces and stars) are provided for each rating scale category in order to augment understanding and enhance the accessibility of the self-report. In addition, a variety of modifications can be made to the administrative procedures to maximize accessibility for children without impacting the reliability of the rating scales (Keller & Kielhofner, 2005). Research has demonstrated that the COSA's two rating scales (competence and value) can be used in a valid and reliable manner by young clients, and the items represent a valid construct of occupational competence and value for occupations (Keller, Kafkes, & Kielhofner, 2005; Keller & Kielhofner, 2005).

For an example of how the COSA can be used in practice and all the COSA items, refer to Case Studies #5 and #7. Figure 4-5 shows an excerpt from the COSA rating form.

PEDIATRIC INTEREST PROFILES

The Pediatric Interest Profiles (PIP) (Henry, 2000) is a self-report that surveys children's and adolescents' play and leisure interests. Three versions within the PIP cover a range of ages, including the Kid Play Profile (KPP) for children ages 6 to 9, the Preteen Play Profile (PPP) for youth 9 to 12, and the Adolescent Leisure Interest Profile (ALIP) for adolescents ages 12 to 21. Responding to a variety of age-appropriate leisure activities, young clients report their level of participation and indicate their feelings of enjoyment associated with the activity. The PIP also asks children to indicate if they do the activities alone or with others. The kid and preteen versions of the PIP use line drawings that represent the various play activities.

Similar to the COSA, the PIP can be used to facilitate a conversation between the child and therapist regarding the child's interests and play needs, build rapport, and maintain a client-centered focus in the therapy process. Total scores for the three versions of the PIP have acceptable test-retest reliability (Henry, 2000). In addition, scores on the ALIP have been found to discriminate between adolescents with and without disabilities (Henry, 1998).

Name:	Day and Time of Evaluation:
Date of Birth:	Date:
Sex: ☐ Male ☐ Female	Session: ☐ I ☐ II

Spaces

Setting in which child was observed: _____

☐ Natural   ☐ Artificial

☐ Indoors   ☐ Outdoors

☐ Quiet   ☐ Noisy

Space for movement: ☐ Small   ☐ Adequate

Additional Factors Influencing Volition:

Objects

☐ Familiar   ☐ Unfamiliar

☐ Natural   ☐ Fabricated

☐ Similar   ☐ Dissimilar

☐ Simple   ☐ Complex

☐ Few   ☐ Many

Additional Factors Influencing Volition:

Social Environment

☐ Individual   ☐ One-to-One

☐ Group: *(Number of individuals)*:_____

☐ Familiar   ☐ Unfamiliar

☐ Peers   ☐ Adults

☐ Chosen by child   ☐ Pre-selected

Additional Factors Influencing Volition:

Occupational Forms

Activity/ies the child is engaged in: _____

☐ Familiar   ☐ Unfamiliar

☐ Structured   ☐ Unstructured

☐ Adequate Challenge   ☐ Inadequate Challenge

☐ Chosen by child   ☐ Pre-selected

Additional Factors Influencing Volition:

Figure 4-6. Environmental form from the PVQ. (Reprinted with permission from the MOHO Clearinghouse, Dept. of Occupational Therapy, University of Illinois at Chicago.)

THE PEDIATRIC VOLITIONAL QUESTIONNAIRE

The PVQ (Basu et al., 2002) is an observational assessment that systematically captures a child's behavior in a variety of environments in order to understand their volition. Developed for young children ages 2 to 6, the PVQ may also be used with older children who are unable to communicate their sense of capacity and interests. When administering the PVQ, the therapist observes the child in at least two different environments, noting the differences in the physical and social environments and considering their impact on the child's volition. The therapist then rates the child on 14 items which range across the continuum of volition (Reilly, 1974): exploration ("shows curiosity"), competency ("stays engaged"), and achievement ("tries to solve problems"). By considering the differences in the child's actions across different environments, the therapist can identify environments that support the development of the child's sense of capacity and effectiveness.

Repeated studies on the PVQ have confirmed the construct validity of the items and demonstrated that they fall along the continuum of volitional development, with the easiest items representing the exploration stage of volitional development and more difficult items representing volitional achievement (Anderson, 1998; Anderson, Kielhofner, & Lai, 2005; Basu, 2003; Geist, 1998). In addition, the PVQ has been determined to be a sensitive measure of a child's volition (Anderson et al., 2005).

For an example of how the PVQ can be used in practice and the view the PVQ items and rating scale, refer to Case Studies #1 and #3. The environmental form used in the PVQ is pictured in Figure 4-6.

THE SHORT CHILD OCCUPATIONAL PROFILE

When clinicians working with children in the Chicago area were looking for a screening tool that would address MOHO concepts, they requested a pediatric version of the Model of Human Occupation Screening Tool, a clinician-developed screening tool used with adults (Parkinson, Forsyth, & Kielhofner, 2004). The SCOPE (Bowyer, Ross, Schwartz, Kielhofner, & Kramer, 2005) uses observation as well as parent report, information from other professionals, and chart reviews to determine if a child's volition, habituation, skills, and environment facilitate or restrict their occupational participation. The SCOPE's flexibility and ease of use allows it to be used as an initial assessment tool as well as an outcome measure. In addition, the scores on the SCOPE provide a visual representation of the strengths of the child and the areas that are problematic. When using the SCOPE, therapists rate each child according to his or her individual developmental trajectory rather than relying on standardized developmental scales, making the SCOPE an occupation- and context-based assessment (Coster, 1998). A recent study confirms that therapists use the SCOPE in a consistent manner and that the SCOPE items make up a valid construct of occupational participation (Bowyer, Kramer, Kielhofner, Barbosa, & Girolami, in press).

For an example of how the SCOPE can be used in practice and to view SCOPE items and rating scale, refer to Case Studies #4 and #7.

THE SCHOOL SETTING INTERVIEW

The SSI (Hemmingsson, Egilson, Hoffman, & Kielhofner, 2005) is a collaborative interview that allows children and adolescents with disabilities to describe the student-environment fit within multiple school settings such as the classroom, playground, gymnasium, and corridors. Through observation, interview, and discussion, the student and therapist work together to identify any needs for accommodations in order to support occupational participation. Sixteen items such as "take exams" and "go on field trips" are also given a rating based on the discussion with the student. Originally developed for students ages 10 and up with physical disabilities, the SSI can also be used with students with developmental and emotional/behavioral disabilities.

The SSI was originally developed in Sweden and has been translated into English. Studies indicate that the SSI demonstrates construct validity (Hemmingsson, Kottorp, & Bernspång, 2004) and has good test-retest reliability (Hemmingsson & Borell, 1996). Research confirms that the SSI effectively identifies students' unmet needs and potential modifications (Borg & Nålsén, 2003; Hemmingsson & Borell, 1996, 2000).

For an example of how the SSI can be used in practice, refer to Case Study #6. The SSI items and rating scale are depicted in Figure 4-7.

SUMMARY

MOHO assessments provide therapists with a means of systematically assessing MOHO concepts such as volition, habituation, skills, and environmental impact. Table 4-3 summarizes the MOHO concepts addressed in each assessment and the administration information.

The four-step rating scale:

4=Perfect fit—when the student perceives that the school-environment fit is ideal and the student does not need any adjustments at all. Thus, the student has no need for adjustments.

3=Good fit—when the student perceives that the school environment has been adapted to meet the student's needs. Thus, the student has received the adjustments needed and is satisfied with the adjustments made.

2=Partial fit—when the student perceives that the school environment needs to be modified but the student has only received some of the adjustment needed. Thus, the student already has some adjustments but perceives that additional adjustment is needed.

1=Unfit—when the student perceives that the school environment needs to be modified but has not received any adjustments at all. Thus, the student needs new adjustments.

Student:

Date:

	Rating steps			
	Perfect fit	Good fit	Partial fit	Unfit
Item	**4**	**3**	**2**	**1**
1.Write				
2.Read				
3.Speak				
4.Remember things				
5.Do mathematics				
6.Do homework				
7.Take exams				
8.Do sports activities				
9.Practical subjects				
10.The classroom				
11.Social break activities				
12.Practical break activit.				
13.Go on field trips				
14.Get assistance				
15.Access the school				
16.Interact with staff				

Figure 4-7. SSI items and rating scale. (Reprinted with permission from the Swedish Association of Occupational Therapists and the MOHO Clearinghouse from Hemmingsson, H., Egilson, S., Hoffman, O., & Kielhofner, G. [2005]. *The School Setting Interview [SSI]* [version 3.0]. Chicago: Swedish Association of Occupational Therapists.)

Table 4-3

MOHO PEDIATRIC AND YOUTH ASSESSMENTS

Assessment	Occupational Adaptation		Volition			Habituation		Environment		Skills			Method of Gathering Data					Target Age	Setting Used
	Identity	Competence	Personal Causation	Interests	Values	Habits	Roles	Physical	Social	Motor	Process	Communication/Interaction	Performance	Participation	Observation	Self-Report	Interview		
Child Occupational Self Assessment (COSA)		X	X	X	X	X	X			X	X	X	X	X		X		8 to 12 years (up to 17)	Community, home health, inpatient, outpatient, school
Pediatric Interest Profiles (PIP)			X	X			X							X		X		6 to 21 years	Community, home health, inpatient, outpatient, school
Pediatric Volitional Questionnaire (PVQ)			X	X	X			X	X						X			2 to 6 years (or older children as appropriate)	Community, home health, inpatient, outpatient, school
Short Child Occupational Profile (SCOPE)			X	X	X	X	X	X	X	X	X	X	X	X	X		X	0 to 21 years	Community, home health, inpatient, outpatient, school
School Setting Interview (SSI)								X	X				X		X		X	10 to 21 years	School

(Adapted from Kielhofner, G. [2004]. Conceptual foundations of occupational therapy [3rd ed., p. 156]. Philadelphia: F.A. Davis Co.)

Case Study #6: Using MOHO-Based Assessments*

Lilja is 13 years old and in eighth grade in her neighborhood school. Lilja sustained a head injury when she was in sixth grade and spent much of the next year in a hospital. Prior to the accident she was a talented student and particularly skillful in crafts and sports. As a result of her accident Lilja's left side is weak. She uses a walker to get around the school premises and a wheelchair for longer trips with the family. Lilja also has visual problems and uses strong glasses. The school occupational therapist, Kristin, decided to administer the SSI and ask Lilja questions about her opportunities to perform and participate in activities in school. Lilja provided the following information:

1. **Write:** Lilja uses a computer for most of her written work in school and at home. She can access the computer herself and operate the software required. Although competent in computer use, Lilja cannot produce classroom work at an adequate speed to keep up with peers, and usually runs into problems in taking notes. She also finds it hard to write and listen to the teacher at the same time.

2. **Read:** Lilja reads about four pages at a time. She can bring out the books she needs and handle them without problem. Lilja transfers her books between classrooms in a basket on her walker and finds it works well.

3. **Speak:** Lilja is not shy of talking in front of class, as she knows all her classmates and the teachers. She raises her hand to answer questions and to call for attention.

4. **Remember things:** Lilja says she forgets her daily schedule very easily. To overcome the problem she tells others what she needs to remember, and they remind her when necessary. Lilja often forgets what to study at home. She would like to use a notepad to write down things she needs to remember, such as her homework.

5. **Do mathematics:** Lilja claims she used to be good at mathematics but that she is not any more. Lilja has different math assignments than most of her classmates. The classroom assistant usually writes up the math problems, and Lilja writes down the answers. Sometimes she does her math on the computer.

6. **Do homework:** Lilja says her homework usually takes about an hour. Occasionally she needs assistance from her parents. She does not write down information about homework from the blackboard, and she cannot always remember what to study at home.

7. **Take exams:** Lilja takes her exams in a special room in school along with another disabled student. A classroom assistant is present and clarifies things if needed. Lilja says she frequently needs more time than allowed. She would prefer to take exams in the early afternoon to be able to concentrate better.

8. **Do sports activities:** Lilja stopped going to gym class after her accident. She is content about this arrangement and does not want to start gym again.

9. **Do practical subjects:** Lilja loves sewing and can use the sewing machine herself. In art she draws what she wants while the other students get specific assignments. The assistant takes Lilja's special chair to art, but not to other practical subject settings such as home economics or crafts. Lilja would prefer to have her chair there as well.

*Case study modified with permission from the Swedish Association of Occupational Therapists and the MOHO Clearinghouse from Hemmingsson, H., Egilson, S., Hoffman, O., & Kielhofner, G. (2005). *The School Setting Interview (SSI)* (version 3.0). Chicago: Swedish Association of Occupational Therapists.

10. **Participate in the classroom:** Lilja sits by the door where there is enough space for the walker. She has a specially adapted chair that she is pleased with. She often has problems getting around the classroom, as the floor is usually cluttered with her classmates' backpacks. Occasionally Lilja gets help to get her books and materials from her backpack, either from her assistant or from her classmates.

11. **Participate in social activities during breaks:** Lilja usually stays inside during breaks and is allowed to have someone with her. Her classmates usually go to a shop near school during breaks. Lilja would like to join them and claims she could if she had her wheelchair at school.

12. **Participate in practical activities at breaks:** Lilja gets assistance in getting her food in the cafeteria as she cannot carry her tray. She is independent in eating and drinking but occasionally needs help to open small containers. She can complete all toileting tasks in school without help or supervision.

13. **Go on field trips:** Lilja takes the wheelchair on field trips. She claims her needs are met most of the time but not always. In a few days her classmates are scheduled to take a trip to the country. Lilja will not join the class on the trip, and she does not know why.

14. **Get assistance:** A class assistant is present during much of Lilja's school day. Lilja likes her assistant. On a few occasions her assistant, Katla, or her other classmates help her out with things. Lilja says the teachers know all about her needs in school and she would not want her fellow students to know any more than they already do.

15. **Access the school:** At wintertime it often gets slippery around the school building. Otherwise, the school building is quite accessible. Although it is on two floors, there is an elevator installed that Lilja manages herself.

16. **Interact with staff:** Lilja is quite content and believes the school staff are knowledgeable about her special needs in school and try to accommodate them when possible.

Following the interview, Lilja and the therapist completed the Intervention Planning form together. In collaboration they determined the type of adjustments needed to improve Lilja's participation in school. An action plan stating the necessary steps and the team members involved was also formed (by whom, when it will be done, where, and how) (Figure 4-8). As many of the goals involved various team members, a meeting was scheduled with Lilja's parents, her teacher, and her assistant to discuss the goals and to ensure that they were realistic and achievable within the timeframe required.

Case Study #6 Learning Activity

1. What MOHO concepts does the SSI primarily assess?
2. What other MOHO concepts does the SSI address?
3. Why do you think the therapist selected the SSI to assess Lilja's situation?
4. What other MOHO assessments would have been appropriate to use to assess Lilja's situation?
5. How would using a different assessment yield different results? How would the intervention plan be changed if another assessment was used?

Item	Environmental Adjustments				Team Members	Steps for Implementation; whom, when, where and how
	Physical		Social			
	Space	Objects	Forms	Groups		
1. Write			Ask the teacher to copy her notes. Otherwise the assistant has to take notes		Lilja, Kristin, teacher and assistant	Kristin discusses the arrangements with teacher and assistant. Lilja will get notes before March 1.
4. Remember things		Notepad	The assistant helps Lilja to write if needed		Lilja, Lilja's parents, Kristin and assistant	Lilja asks her parents to buy her a notepad before March 1. Kristin discusses the arrangement with the assistant.
7. Take exams			Extended time during examinations. If possible, schedule exams to suit Lilja		Lilja, Kristin, principal and teacher	Kristin discusses the arrangements with the principal and teacher.
9. Do practical subjects		Special chair in crafts and home management			Lilja, Kristin and assistant	Kristin brings up the question with the assistant. Measures should be taken before March 1.
10. Participate in the classroom				Ask the classmates not to leave their backpacks on the floor	Lilja, classmates, Kristin and teacher	Lilja brings up the subject with her classmates before March 1. Kristin discusses the arrangement with Lilja's teacher.
11. Participate in social break activities	Lilja needs a wheelchair in school for use during breaks				Lilja, Kristin, Lilja's parents, teacher and assistant	Lilja discusses with her parents whether or not it is possible to bring her wheelchair to school on a daily basis. Otherwise Kristin explores the possibilities of ordering a new wheelchair to keep in school.
13. Go on field trips				Discuss the practical aspects of planning field trips that also suit Lilja	Kristin, teacher, principal and Lilja	Kristin discusses the practical aspects of field trip planning with the principal and teacher so Lilja can participate in the spring and onwards.

Figure 4-8. Lilja's action plan using the SSI. (Reprinted with permission from the Swedish Association of Occupational Therapists and the MOHO Clearinghouse from Hemmingsson, H., Egilson, S., Hoffman, O., & Kielhofner, G. [2005]. *The School Setting Interview [SSI]* [version 3.0]. Chicago: Swedish Association of Occupational Therapists.)

— SECTION VI —

Model of Human Occupation in the Literature

USING THE MODEL OF HUMAN OCCUPATION IN PRACTICE: INTERVENTIONS AND PROGRAMS

MOHO has been used to develop intervention programs for children and youth for the past 20 years. MOHO provides an appropriate framework for programming and facilitates children's occupational adaptation since it explains how problems with occupational adaptation occur and outlines the mechanism required for change (Braveman, Kielhofner, Belanger, de las Heras, & Llerena, 2002).

MOHO has been used most often by therapists working with children and adolescents in mental health, and this application has proven to be international. Adelstein and her colleagues (1989) and Baron (1987, 1989, 1991) demonstrated how MOHO could be applied in child and adolescent psychiatry. For example, the activities required to run a youth-published newspaper were aligned with the stages of volitional development and included brainstorming new ideas for stories, following through with writing assignments, and sitting on the editorial board (Baron, 1987). Other program ideas like hobby clubs, workshops, play fairs, and home economics (Baron, 1989, 1991; Weissenberg & Giladi, 1989) have been used to support young people's acquisition of new interests, facilitate more effective habits and routines, and increase clients' sense of competence.

Services for youth with chemical dependency have focused on the development of self-esteem and work roles using MOHO as a guiding model (Scarth, 1983). In Belgium, a program based on MOHO was developed for a children's ward in a psychiatric hospital (Reekmans & Kielhofner, 1998). The intervention focused on the supports and resources available in the environment and recognized occupation as a mechanism for change. In the United Kingdom, in response to a recent conference of occupational therapists working in child and adolescent mental health, Harrison and Forsyth (2005) called for the use of MOHO in mental health settings in order to provide child-centered and occupation-focused service.

MOHO has also been used with children and adolescents in other types of occupational therapy service provision. In one case involving a child who was diagnosed with attention deficit hyperactivity disorder, compensatory strategies were used to increase functional performance; the development of personal causation, interests, and values were considered an outcome of improved performance (Woodrum, 1993). An occupational therapy intervention based on MOHO was designed to address the psychosocial needs of an adolescent with insulin-dependent diabetes mellitus (Curtin, 1991). Schaff and Mulrooney (1989) proposed a family-centered approach to early intervention services that combined MOHO with developmental perspectives of play. This early intervention approach focused on the MOHO concepts of volition, habituation, and skill in order to address the child's and parent's needs.

Occupational therapists have also found MOHO to be useful when working with youth in the community. Therapists addressed the needs of Mayan Indian children, adolescents, and their families who returned to Guatemala after 14 years as refuges in Mexico by creating a community program based on MOHO (Simo-Algado & Cardona, 2005). This program had a strong focus on the cultural aspects of environment and its influence on occupational adaptation. In another community-based program serving children survivors of the Kosovo conflict, MOHO was used to guide identification of occupational performance problems (Simo-Algado, Mehta, Kronenberg, Cockburn, & Kirsh, 2002). Finally, MOHO concepts guided an intervention that enabled street children to write and perform plays in order to develop new interests and experience new social groups and occupational forms/tasks (Kronenberg, 1999).

Learning Activity I

1. Describe the settings where MOHO has been systematically implemented in the occupational therapy process.
2. Describe how MOHO could be systematically implemented during evaluation, intervention, and outcomes at a pediatric occupational therapy setting you are familiar with.

Case Study #7: MOHO Programs

By Bridget Caruso, OTR/L

Bright colored pictures, butterflies on the ceiling, video games, musicians and clowns, art projects, and parties...sounds like an ideal vacation spot for children. However, this picture is actually an acute care pediatric floor in an inner city hospital. The parties are for children going home after a transplant, for a little girl spending her 6th birthday in the hospital because she is in her second round of chemotherapy, and for an 18-year-old young man graduating from high school despite his many admissions to the hospital related to sickle cell anemia. The butterflies on the ceiling are for the children who lie in bed recovering from heart surgery, brain surgery, or orthopedic surgery. The video games are for kids who cannot leave their room because they are isolated due to precautions for infections. The clowns and musicians bring smiles to the children while they spend years of their lives surrounded by doctors, nurses, and therapists.

This inner city acute care team includes occupational therapy. The team not only treats children with cancer, but also educates families and interdisciplinary staff on the importance of occupations and client-centered care. Establishing a client-centered framework in this acute care pediatric ward is supported by the implementation of MOHO across disciplines through guidance from the occupational therapist. The components of MOHO help to shape a client-centered treatment plan and establish a continuum of development in and out of the hospital. This is accomplished by educating staff members, incorporating MOHO language in staff meetings and documentation, and recognizing each individual child's and family's roles, interests, and habits both in the hospital and at home.

The incorporation of MOHO concepts such as habits, roles, values, motivation (volition), and environment into bedside rounds, discharge planning, and parent education sessions did not happen overnight. The occupational therapist first began using MOHO language in documentation and when communicating with the doctors, nurses, and families. The occupational therapist demonstrated how the use of MOHO identified child and family values that directly influenced the choices made during hospital stays, in rehabilitation, and when managing health once discharged. Once interdisciplinary staff supervisors began to recognize the benefit of gaining a more holistic picture of each child and his or her family, they endorsed the unit-wide implementation of MOHO concepts. Since the hospital is a teaching facility, new residents participate in in-service seminars on MOHO and occupational performance. They are provided with an overview of the theory, but more importantly receive support and guidance from the therapist on how to incorporate MOHO concepts into treatment planning. The residents are familiar with the terminology and are beginning to identify each child and his or her family's needs and interests. Resident feedback indicates that this has been viewed as a learning experience and expanded their domain of care from medical pathology to the physical and emotional well-being of the child and his or her family. Identifying the importance of volition, routines, habits, interests, and recognizing the roles that these children both give up and take on while in the hospital has become second nature for the medical team.

Occupational performance is assessed in this population with tools based on MOHO, such as the COSA and SCOPE. These assessment tools also help to identify loss of occupational performance that may not be noted on traditional medical admissions. The assessment results may reveal changes in client motivation, his or her environment, or his or her routine that is impacting his or her overall wellness and ability to manage his or her health. In addition, the outcomes of these assessments provide information to the interdisciplinary team that enables them to incorporate a more client-centered plan of care.

Incorporating a client-centered approach may be as simple as setting up a daily routine and monitoring role performance. For example, during a 15-year-old female's prolonged stay at the hospital for chemotherapy, nurses noted that she stopped getting dressed and stayed in her room for long periods throughout the day. The change in her routine and lack of motivation to participate in self-care enabled the staff to identify a decrease in role performance. Using this terminology, they requested that the occupational therapist help monitor and identify changes in motivation and her corresponding rehabilitation success. The occupational therapist used the COSA with the young lady to better understand her motivation for doing self-care activities. The client's responses began a discussion where she shared that she preferred to wear her street clothes when in the hospital instead of the hospital gown. She also identified the importance of wearing her wig and make-up before going to the playroom or going to therapy sessions out of her room. The occupational therapist worked with the young lady and nursing staff to set aside time in her routine for "looking good." As a result, the young lady began to leave her room more often during free time and had better attendance at therapy sessions.

The SCOPE is another MOHO tool that has been useful for parent education. The use of the SCOPE as a parent interview allows parents to express strengths, difficulties, and expectations of their child during the hospital stay. Allowing the parents to communicate a prehospitalization picture of their child also gives a baseline of performance when planning intervention activities. For example, following a surgical procedure and an extended period of hospitalization, a 10-year-old nonverbal little boy with cerebral palsy refused to eat. The team was concerned about dehydration and malnutrition and began to consider alternative feeding measures. During the occupational therapist's initial assessment, which included the administration of the SCOPE as a parent interview, the mother identified that at home her son was independent in feeding and had his own way of communicating when he was hungry. She also shared that at home he had compensatory mobility strategies and moved independently from room to room. He also engaged in leisure activities independently and enjoyed social interactions with family members. The current hospital environment did not support his compensatory communication and mobility, and its restrictive schedule did not allow him to actively participate in more natural mealtime routines and eating habits. The loss of his familiar routine led to his withdrawal from social and leisure activities following surgery and resulted in his refusal to participate in therapy and eating. The hospital team was able to better address these global issues following the occupational therapy initial evaluation. Changes were made to support the child in regaining some control, and he began to make choices during mealtime and had improved motivation for eating. At time of discharge the child had begun to gain weight and was working to regain his mobility strategies.

The occupational therapist not only considers the needs of the child, but also their family's needs. Within the hospital community, parents experience changes in their roles (acquiring the role of parenting a sick and sometimes dying child) and encounter shifts in the family's routines and traditions. Sometimes parents have difficulty identifying new roles and ways to enact those roles. For instance, if a baby is unable to breast/bottle feed due to medical contraindications, a new mother may be frustrated by not being able to care for her child in this way. She may benefit from a parent session with the occupational therapist to demonstrate other ways to implement caregiving and bonding routines with her new baby, such as kangaroo care and through provision of non-nutritive oral stimulation to her infant. This not only supports the mother's occupational identity as a parent, but facilitates the baby's developmental and self-regulatory skills. The outcome of these interactions may improve family dynamics, prevent depression or withdrawal from parenting, empower the family when speaking with the medical team, and prepare the family for the discharge of their child.

MOHO concepts used in this acute care setting create a "universal" occupational language and an occupational focus for the entire medical team that helps bring a child and his or her family's face to a medical record number. Using this framework has helped the pediatric floor become more client- and family-centered and holistically oriented, as interests, values, roles, and environmental supports are as common in everyday language as antibiotics, precautions, and diagnoses.

Case Study #7 Learning Activity

How are MOHO concepts used in this acute ward?
- In evaluation?
- In intervention?
- In evaluating outcomes?

MODEL OF HUMAN OCCUPATION-BASED RESEARCH WITH CHILDREN AND YOUTH

In addition to the research conducted to develop psychometrically sound MOHO-based assessments, other research supports the application of MOHO with young clients and their families.

Several studies have demonstrated that MOHO concepts manifest themselves differently in young individuals with mental health problems as compared to young persons without identified mental health problems. An early study using MOHO demonstrated that adolescents who had psychosocial difficulties differed from adolescents without difficulties on measures of personal causation (Smyntek, Barris, & Kielhofner, 1985). Barris and colleagues (1986) found that a sense of competence, the perceived importance of daily activities, and the number of valued roles discriminated between three groups of adolescents: those with psychological illness, those with a psychiatric diagnosis, and those without any identified mental health problems. Several years later a study that included adolescent psychiatric clients had similar findings, as those with mental health problems differed from individuals without a psychiatric diagnosis on measures of personal and environmental characteristics (Barris, Dickie, & Baron, 1988). Finally, the number of current and future anticipated roles and the presence of strong interests were found to discriminate between adolescent males with and without psychosocial difficulties (Ebb, Coster, & Duncombe, 1989).

Attempting to determine the factors related to symptom management and functioning 6 months after a young person's first experience of a psychotic disorder, Henry (1994) found that several MOHO concepts were related to good outcomes and occupational participation. In addition to gender, duration of symptom onset, and age of onset (Henry, 1994; Henry & Coster, 1996), the presence of roles prior to and after onset and overall occupational adaptation were significant predictors of better global functioning 6 months after onset. A strong interest in recreational activities and a positive perception of social competence were also predictive of occupational adaptation (Henry, 1994; Henry & Coster, 1996).

These studies reveal the impact that interests, self-perceptions, and roles have on young people with mental health difficulties. Therapists working with clients with these needs should facilitate their discovery of and participation in a variety of occupations that they find interesting and valuable and identify environments that support future occupational adaptation.

Several other studies conducted with children and youth in a variety of settings have used MOHO as a framework for data collection or analysis. A pilot study conducted with six adolescents in a correctional facility sought to examine the effect of participation in craft occupations such as leatherworking, woodworking, and clay (DeForest, Watts, &

Madigan, 1991). Researchers found that participation led to an increase of skills, which then enhanced the adolescents' sense of capacity. When trying to better understand how youth with hemiplegic cerebral palsy experienced various occupations, Skoid, Josephsson, and Eliasson (2004) used MOHO ideas of performance to guide the group interviews and data analysis. Finally, Jacobson's (2003) qualitative study of children diagnosed with autism in inclusionary classrooms explored the factors that led to their participation as class members. Physical space such as seating arrangements of children with and without disabilities, the presence of personal belongings in the classroom, participation in classroom activities and group work, and mutual relationships in which students held each other accountable led to increased participation and the recognition of students with autism as genuine members of the classroom community.

Learning Activity J

1. List the MOHO concepts that discriminate between adolescents identified as having mental health and psychosocial difficulties and those who do not.
2. What MOHO concepts predict occupational participation 6 months after onset of a young person's first psychotic experience?

SUMMARY

The literature demonstrates how MOHO can be used with children and adolescents in a variety of settings including inpatient psychiatry, early intervention, and community-based service provision. The research findings point to the importance of addressing the MOHO concepts of personal causation, interests, roles, habits, and the social and physical environment when working with children and youth. These findings provide the evidence to support the application of MOHO in the evaluation and intervention with young clients.

Conclusion

Using MOHO concepts, therapeutic reasoning, and assessment tools allows a therapist to systematically consider, assess, and document concepts essential to occupational adaptation. Through MOHO, therapists are able to identify and focus in on the strengths that children possess and identify ways to enhance those strengths in the child's environment. MOHO uses the concepts of volition, habituation, performance capacity, and the environment to understand a child's participation in occupations and the context within which activity occurs. By using MOHO in practice, therapists are able to focus on individual needs that affect occupational participation rather than on specific physical or cognitive limitations.

Most models that are used in pediatric practice are developmentally based and place a heavy emphasis on a child's impairments. MOHO shifts therapists from viewing the limitations children have to the strengths that exist and then taps into those strengths to improve overall occupational participation. Through MOHO, therapists are able to begin to view each child individually, gain a better understanding of a child's occupational participation, and tap into a child's motivation to participate in occupations.

Because MOHO shifts attention from impairment to occupational participation, families can better understand the abilities of their child and identify ways to enhance their child's ability to derive satisfaction in activities. This conceptual basis for occupational therapy intervention can give children and their families hope while tapping into the needs of the child and the family within the environment that the child lives.

References

Adelstein, L. A., Barnes, M. A., Murray-Jensen, F., & Skaggs, C. B. (1989). A broadening frontier: Occupational therapy in mental health programs for children and adolescents. *Mental Health Special Interest Section Newsletter, 12,* 2-4.

American Occupational Therapy Association. (2002). Occupational therapy practice framework: Domain and process. *American Journal of Occupational Therapy, 56,* 609-639.

Anderson, S. P. (1998*). Using the Pediatric Volitional Questionnaire to assess children with disabilities* [unpublished master's thesis]. University of Illinois at Chicago, Chicago, IL.

Anderson, S., Kielhofner, G., & Lai, J. S. (2005). An examination of the measurement properties of the pediatric volitional questionnaire. *Physical and Occupational Therapy in Pediatrics, 25,* 39-57.

Bandura, A., Barbaranelli, C., Caprara, G. V., & Pastorelli, C. (1996). Multifaceted impact of self-efficacy beliefs on academic functioning. *Child Development, 67,* 1206-1222.

Baron, K. (1987). The model of human occupation: A newspaper treatment group for adolescents with a diagnosis of conduct disorder. *Occupational Therapy in Mental Health, 7*(2), 89-104.

Baron, K. (1989). Occupational therapy: A program for child psychiatry. *Mental Health Special Interest Section Newsletter, 12,* 6-7.

Baron, K. B. (1991). The use of play in child psychiatry: Reframing the therapeutic environment. *Occupational Therapy in Mental Health, 11*(2/3), 37-56.

Barris, R., Dickie, V., & Baron, K. (1988). A comparison of psychiatric patients and normal subjects based on the Model of Human Occupation. *Occupational Therapy Journal of Research, 8,* 3-37.

Barris, R., Kielhofner, G., Burch, R. M., Gelinas, I., Klement, M., & Schultz, B. (1986). Occupational function and dysfunction in three groups of adolescents. *Occupational Therapy Journal of Research, 6,* 301-317.

Basu, S. (2003). *Measurement properties of the Pediatric Volitional Questionnaire* [unpublished master's thesis]. University of Illinois at Chicago, Chicago, IL.

Basu, B., Kafkes, A., Geist, R., & Kielhofner, G. (2002). *The Pediatric Volitional Questionnaire (PVQ)* (version 2.0). Model of Human Occupation Clearinghouse, Department of Occupational Therapy, College of Applied Health Sciences, University of Illinois at Chicago, Chicago, IL.

Beery, K. E., Buktenica, N. A., & Beery, N. A. (2004). *The Beery-Buktenica Developmental Test of Visual-Motor Integration.* Minneapolis, MN: NCS Pearson, Inc.

Borg, G., & Nålsén, H. (2003). *Validitetsprövning av instrumentet Bedömning av anpassningar i skolmiljön (BAS). Mäter BAS behovet av anpassningar i skolmiljön?* (translated: Validation of the School Setting Interview. Does the SSI measure the need for adjustments in the school setting?) Stockholm: Neurotec, Karolinska Institutet.

Bowyer, P., Kramer, J., Kielhofner, G., Barbosa, V., & Girolami, G. (in press). The measurement properties of the Short Child Occupational Profile (SCOPE). *Physical and Occupational Therapy in Pediatrics.*

Bowyer, P., Ross, M., Schwartz, O., Kielhofner, G., & Kramer, J. (2005). *The Short Child Occupational Profile (SCOPE)* (version 2.1). Model of Human Occupation Clearinghouse, Department of Occupational Therapy, College of Applied Health Sciences, University of Illinois at Chicago, Chicago, IL.

Braveman, B., Kielhofner, G., Belanger, R., de las Heras, G., & Llerena, V. (2002). Program development. In G. Kielhofner (Ed.), *Model of Human Occupation: Theory and application* (3rd ed., pp. 491-519). Baltimore: Lippincott, Williams & Wilkins.

Coster, W. (1998). Occupation-centered assessment of children. *American Journal of Occupational Therapy, 52,* 337-344.

Curtin, C. (1991). Psychosocial intervention with an adolescent with diabetes using the model of human occupation. *Occupational Therapy in Mental Health 11*(2/3), 23-36.

DeForest, D., Watts, J. H., & Madigan, M. J. (1991). Resonation in the model of human occupation: A pilot study. *Occupational Therapy in Mental Health, 11*(2/3), 57-75.

Ebb, E. W., Coster, W. J., & Duncombe, L. (1989). Comparison of normal and psychosocially dysfunctional male adolescents. *Occupational Therapy in Mental Health, 9*(2), 53-74.

Fisher, A. (1999). *Assessment of motor and process skills* (3rd ed.). Ft. Collins, CO: Three Star Press.

Folio, M. R. & Fewell, R. R. (2000). *Peabody Developmental Motor Scales (PDMS-2)* (2nd ed.). Hingham, MA: Teaching Resources.

Forsyth, K., & Kielhofner, G. (1999). Validity of the assessment of communication and interaction skills. *British Journal of Occupational Therapy, 62,* 69-74.

Geist, R. (1998). *The validity study of the Pediatric Volitional Questionnaire* [unpublished master's thesis]. University of Illinois at Chicago, Chicago, IL.

Gill, C. (1997). Four types of integration in disability identity development. *Journal of Vocational Rehabilitation, 9,* 39-46.

Hammel, J., Finlayson, M., Kielhofner, G., Helfrich, C., & Peterson, L. (2002). Educating scholars of practice: An approach to preparing tomorrow's researchers. *Occupational Therapy in Health Care, 15* (1&2), 157-176.

Harrison, M., & Forsyth, K. (2005). Developing a vision for therapists working within child and adolescent mental health services: Poised or paused for action? *British Journal of Occupational Therapy, 68,* 1-5.

Hemmingsson, H., & Borell, L. (1996). The development of an assessment of adjustment needs in the school setting for use with physically disabled students. *Scandinavian Journal of Occupational Therapy, 3,* 156-162.

Hemmingsson, H., & Borell, L. (2000). Accommodation needs and student-environment fit in upper secondary school for students with severe physical disabilities. *Canadian Journal of Occupational Therapy, 67,* 162-173.

Hemmingsson, H., Egilson, S., Hoffman, O., & Kielhofner, G. (2005). *The School Setting Interview (SSI)* (version 3.0). Chicago: Swedish Association of Occupational Therapists.

Hemmingsson, H., Kottorp, A., & Bernspång, B. (2004). Validity of the school setting interview: An assessment of the student-environment fit. *Scandinavian Journal of Occupational Therapy, 11,* 171-178.

Henry, A. (1994). *Predicting psychosocial functioning and symptomatic recovery of adolescents and young adults with a first psychotic episode: A six-month follow-up study* [doctoral dissertation]. Boston University, Boston, MA.

Henry, A. D. (1998). Development of a measure of adolescent leisure interests. *American Journal of Occupational Therapy, 52,* 531-539.

Henry, A. D. (2000). *The Pediatric Interest Profiles: Surveys of play for children and adolescents.* Available at: www.moho.uic.edu.

Henry, A. D., & Coster, W. J. (1996). Predictors of functional outcome among adolescents and young adults with psychotic disorders. *American Journal of Occupational Therapy, 50*(3), 171-183.

Jacobson, L. (2003). *Fostering participation in the inclusion classroom: A study of elementary school students with autism* [unpublished master's thesis]. University of Illinois at Chicago, Chicago, IL.

Keller, J., Kafkes, A., Basu, S., Federico, J., & Kielhofner, G. (2005). *The Child Occupational Self Assessment (version 2.1).* Model of Human Occupation Clearinghouse, Department of Occupational Therapy, College of Applied Health Sciences, University of Illinois at Chicago, Chicago, IL.

Keller, J., Kafkes, A., & Kielhofner, G. (2005). Psychometric characteristics of the Child Occupational Self Assessment (COSA). Part one: An initial examination of psychometric properties. *Scandinavian Journal of Occupational Therapy, 12*(3), 118-127.

Keller, J., & Kielhofner, G. (2005). Psychometric characteristics of the Child Occupational Self Assessment (COSA). Part two: Refining the psychometric properties. *Scandinavian Journal of Occupational Therapy, 12*(4), 147-158.

Kielhofner, G. (2004). *Conceptual foundations of occupational therapy* (3rd ed.). Philadelphia: F.A. Davis Co.

Kielhofner, G. (2005). Scholarship and practice: Bridging the divide. *American Journal of Occupational Therapy, 59*(2), 231-239.

Kielhofner, G. (2007). *The model of human occupation: Theory and application* (4th ed.). Baltimore: Lippincott, Williams & Wilkins.

Kronenberg, F. C. W. (1999). *Street children: Being and becoming.* Hogeschool Limburg, Heerlen, the Netherlands.

Linton, S. (1998). Disability studies/not disability studies. In S. Linton (Ed.), *Claiming disability: Knowledge and identity* (pp. 132-156). New York: University Press.

Longmore, P. K. (2003). *Why I burned my book and other essays on disability.* Philadelphia: Temple University Press.

Oliver, M. (1996). The social model in context. In M. Oliver (Ed.), *Understanding disability from theory to practice* (pp. 30-42). New York: St. Martin's Press.

Parkinson, S., Forsyth, K., & Kielhofner, G. (2004). *The Model of Human Occupation Screening Tool (MOHOST)* (version 2.1). Model of Human Occupation Clearinghouse, Department of Occupational Therapy, College of Applied Health Sciences, University of Illinois at Chicago, Chicago, IL.

Reekmans, M., & Kielhofner, G. (1998). Defining occupational therapy services in child psychiatry: An application of the Model of Human Occupation. *Ergotherapie, 5,* 6-11.

Reilly, M. (1974). *Play as exploratory learning.* Beverly Hills, CA: Sage Publications.

Scarth, P. P. (1983). Services for chemically dependent adolescents. *Mental Health Special Interest Section Newsletter 13,* 7-8.

Schaff, R. C., & Mulrooney, L. L. (1989). Occupational therapy in early intervention: A family-centered approach. *American Journal of Occupational Therapy, 43*(11), 745-754.

Shapiro, J. P. (1993). *No pity: People with disabilities forging a new civil rights movement.* New York: Times Books/ Random House.

Simo-Algado, S., & Cardona, C. E. (2005). The return of the corn men. In F. Kronenberg, S. Simo-Algado, & N. Pollard (Eds.), *Occupational therapy without borders: Learning from the spirit of survivors* (pp. 336-350). United Kingdom: Churchill Livingstone.

Simo-Algado, S., Mehta, N., Kronenberg, F., Cockburn, L., & Kirsh, B. (2002). Occupational therapy intervention with children survivor of war. *Canadian Journal of Occupational Therapy, 69*(4), 205-217.

Skoid, A., Josephsson, S., & Eliasson, A. (2004). Performing bimanual activities: The experiences of young persons with hemiplegic cerebral palsy. *American Journal of Occupational Therapy, 58*(4), 416-425.

Smyntek, L., Barris, R., & Kielhofner, G. (1985). The Model of Human Occupation applied to psychosocially functional and dysfunctional adolescents. *Occupational Therapy in Mental Health, 5*(1), 21-40.

Swain, J., Finkelstein, V., French, S., & Oliver, M. (1993). *Disabling barriers–Enabling environments.* London: Sage.

Wehmeyer, M. L., Kelchner, K., & Richards, S. (1996). Essential characteristics of self determined behavior of individuals with mental retardation. *American Journal on Mental Retardation, 100*(6), 632-642.

Weissenberg, R., & Giladi, N. (1989). Home economics day: A program for disturbed adolescents to promote acquisition of habits and skills. *Occupational Therapy in Mental Health, 9*(2), 89-103.

Wilbarger, P., & Wilbarger, J. (1991). *Sensory defensiveness in children aged 2-12: An intervention guide for parents and other caretakers.* Santa Barbara, CA: Avanti Educational Programs.

Woodrum, S. C. (1993). A treatment approach for attention deficit hyperactivity disorder using the Model of Human Occupation. *Developmental Disabilities Special Interest Section Newsletter, 16*(1), 1-2.

World Health Organization. (2001). *International classification of functioning, disability, and health.* Geneva, Switzerland: Author.

The Occupational Adaptation Model: Application to Child and Family Interventions

Beth Werner DeGrace, PhD, OTR/L

Learning Objectives

At the end of this chapter, the reader will be able to:
- Describe the process of Occupational Adaptation (OA).
- Understand and apply OA as a model.
- Describe the relationship between the OA and the *Occupational Therapy Practice Framework*.
- Analyze case studies to identify the process of OA and dysadaptation and make recommendations for assessment and intervention.

— Section I —

Introduction

Occupational therapy practitioners depend upon models to guide their thinking as they make decisions about what strategies, supports, and intervention methods will be most helpful for supporting children and their families to engage in meaningful life occupations. Occupational Adaptation (OA) can be used as a model to guide professional reasoning and understand how children and their families adapt to and master the occupational challenges associated with everyday living. When used as a model, OA identifies how we, as occupational therapists, can support children and their families to experience relative mastery in their occupational lives.

Introduction to Occupational Adaptation

During the development of a PhD program in occupational therapy at Texas Woman's University, the theory of OA evolved and was introduced in writing in 1992 (Schkade

& Schultz, 1992; Schultz & Schkade, 1992). Since that time numerous research and practice-related publications have emerged (Garrett & Schkade, 1995; Gibson & Schkade, 1997; Hamilton, 2001; Schkade, 1999; Schkade & Schultz, 2003; Schultz, 1997; Schultz & Schkade, 1994, 1997). A book titled *Occupational Adaptation in Practice: Concepts and Cases* has been written and provides an in-depth description of the model with case examples illustrating the process of OA (Schkade & McClung, 2001).

When used as a model, OA provides a means for explaining the interaction between the person and the occupational environment. It provides a way to examine whether or not a person generates, evaluates, and integrates adaptive responses to an occupational challenge and experiences relative mastery. Person can be an individual, such as a child or parent. Person can also be representative of a system, such as family, since a family can have a collective and shared experience of occupation (Werner, 2001). For the purposes of this chapter, person will also imply child, parent, or family.

Occupation and Adaptation Defined

The OA model includes the definition of *occupations* as "those activities in which the individual has active involvement; experiences personal meaning; and engages in a process that yields a product, either tangible or intangible" (Schultz, 1996, p. 6). *Adaptation* is viewed as a response to master challenges. The experience and engagement in adaptation is a normative and universal process, which occurs within the person or family. The need for adaptation is most prominent during periods of life transition.

Basics of the Model

The three basic elements of the process of OA include the person (child, parent, or family), the occupational environment, and the interaction of the two as they come together to afford occupation. Each person brings a desire for mastery in occupation and the occupation is produced within an environment that includes expectations or demands for mastery. As the person and environment interact, there is a press or a definition given to how the occupation will be mastered as evaluated by the person and by the environment. This interaction is the source for occupational performance.

As a person engages in occupation a process of adaptation follows. Because engagement in occupation is a continual and dynamic process, adaptation becomes crucial to occupational performance and the experience of relative mastery. So the interplay between the person, environment, and ensuing challenge necessitates an internal adaptation response, which results in an occupational response and ultimately occupational growth (Figure 5-1).

Our role as occupational therapists is to understand how people engage in the adaptation processes, particularly those that compromise health and well-being. Therefore OA provides a way for understanding: 1) the demands of the occupational environment, 2) the preferences of the person (child, parent, or family), 3) the actions and behaviors generated by a person (child, parent, or family), and 4) how the person (child, parent, or family) and the environment respond to the adaptation that has transpired. These concepts will be explained in greater detail in the following paragraphs.

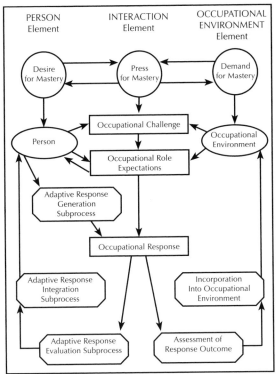

Figure 5-1. Occupational Adaptation. (Republished with permission of the American Occupational Therapy Association, from Occupational adaptation: Toward a holistic approach to contemporary practice, part 1. *American Journal of Occupational Therapy.* J. K. Schkade & S. Schultz, Vol. 46, 1992; permission conveyed through Copyright Clearance Center, Inc.)

Think about who you are today.
1. What are some of your current occupations?
2. Select one of these occupations and identify *why* you are engaging in this occupation and the associated occupational role.
3. Now think about what the environment expects of you as you engage in this occupation role.
4. Does the environment have expectations for how you should behave, act, dress, and/or interact with others?

Expanding Upon Concepts

PERSON

The person is composed of three constants. These constants include the sensorimotor, the cognitive, and the psychosocial elements. Each of these elements is influenced by the genetic, environmental, and experiential/phenomenological aspects of our being or the system's being. When working with children and families it is important to understand how they view occupational role expectations and generate adaptive responses. Collectively, by understanding the person according to the elements described in OA, an understanding of personal preferences and ways of coping/responding to an occupational challenge will be discovered (Figure 5-2).

Figure 5-2. Person element. (Republished with permission of the American Occupational Therapy Association, from Occupational adaptation: Toward a holistic approach to contemporary practice, part 1. *American Journal of Occupational Therapy.* J. K. Schkade & S. Schultz, Vol. 46, 1992; permission conveyed through Copyright Clearance Center, Inc.)

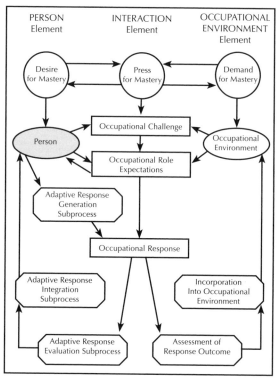

Here are a few ways of thinking about the person elements. Think of a body of water, such as a lake. Some individuals would think what a lovely place to read a book (cognitive) while others would think what a lovely place to swim (sensorimotor). Likewise, how people adapt to stressful situations is also influenced by person elements. For example, if you just found out terrible news some would call a friend (psychosocial) while others would go do an activity (sensorimotor). The following learning activities will encourage you to think about how your occupational being is influenced by your person elements.

Learning Activity B

1. It is important to gain insight into your person or family elements. Think about:
    *   How do you prefer to spend your time?
    *   How do you tackle a new task, such as learning how to put together a bicycle from its parts?
    *   How does your family spend time together?
    *   How does your family share holidays or special celebrations?
    *   What does your family do on the weekends? Weekdays?
    *   How did or does your family handle stressful situations? What roles does each member assume? What does each member do?
2. Relate these aspects to children and families.
    *   How do we identify the preferences of children with severe disabilities?
    *   How do we identify how children with disabilities solve problems?
    *   How do we identify a family's preferred ways of living and coping?

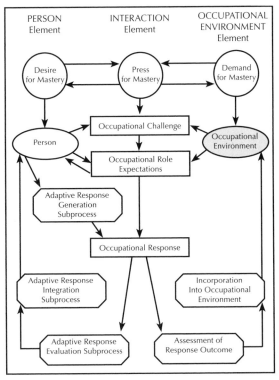

Figure 5-3. Occupational environment element. (Republished with permission of the American Occupational Therapy Association, from Occupational adaptation: Toward a holistic approach to contemporary practice, part 1. *American Journal of Occupational Therapy.* J. K. Schkade & S. Schultz, Vol. 46, 1992; permission conveyed through Copyright Clearance Center, Inc.)

ENVIRONMENT

The environment is where occupation occurs. Similar to the *Occupational Therapy Practice Framework* (American Occupational Therapy Association [AOTA], 2002), the environment (context) for occupation has been identified as the physical, social, and cultural contexts. We perform occupations within leisure, work, or play environments. Each environment has characteristics or subsystems that influence how engagement in occupation is executed. OA defines these subsystems as physical, social, and cultural. Collectively, these give shape to and influence occupational roles.

The physical characteristics are familiar to occupational therapy practitioners and include the tangible aspects of the environment such as lighting, arrangement of furniture, accessibility to a building, and temperature. Social elements include the availability for relationships or the number of individuals and characteristics of the individuals in the environment. Consider a child in elementary school. What is the ratio between adults and children? Are there more adults than children? Are the children verbal or nonverbal? The cultural aspects of the environment include the values, beliefs, attitudes, and expectations of the setting or individuals within the setting. For example, what are the rules of the classroom and school (Figure 5-3)?

1. It is important to now gain insight into the subsystems of the environment. Think about:

   - Going to work during "off" hours, such as the weekend, early in the morning, or late at night. How did the physical, social, and cultural expectations differ from what you know as "work"?

2. Relate this to intervention with children and families.

   - What types of settings do children with severe disabilities spend most of their time? How could this affect their occupational growth and performance?

   - What kinds of expectations exist for children with disabilities? Do they differ from children without disabilities? Does our society expect children with disabilities to go to college or drive a car?

   - How do our cities, childcare facilities, recreational facilities, churches, public buildings, and private buildings support children with disabilities?

     ◦ Think about children with powered mobility or children who use pictures to communicate.

     ◦ Think about children who do not use assistive technology—how do the subsystems of the environment influence occupational performance for children with spastic cerebral palsy, autism, a visual impairment, or a hearing impairment?

   - Given the same environments as above, how do subsystems of the environment support the families of children with disabilities?

OCCUPATIONAL CHALLENGE

An occupational challenge results from the interaction of the person and his or her desire for mastery and the occupational environment and its demand for mastery. Occupational challenges are embedded in the individual's interpretation of the occupational environment and his or her respective role and transpire within an occupational role (Figure 5-4).

Occupational challenges occur constantly within our lives, and generally do not interfere with our ability to fulfill our occupations. One of the main reasons we are in the lives of the children and families is the difficulty they experience in mastering their occupational challenges. This requires occupational therapy practitioners to become skilled at understanding the process of adaptation for the person.

Process of Adaptation

A person generates an adaptive response process when confronted with an occupational challenge. This begins the cycle of adaptation. The process includes generation, evaluation, and integration of an adaptive response. The generation of an adaptive response depends upon two things: mechanisms for adaptation and the adaptation gestalt. The adaptive responses are viewed as elicited and internal, rather than as a taught skill or a rigid pattern of behavior. The successful process of adaptation is necessary for constructing and engaging in occupations that are satisfying, enduring, and fulfilling to the person and/or family. The generation of adaptation responses depends upon these mechanisms of adaptation: energy, modes, and behaviors (Figure 5-5).

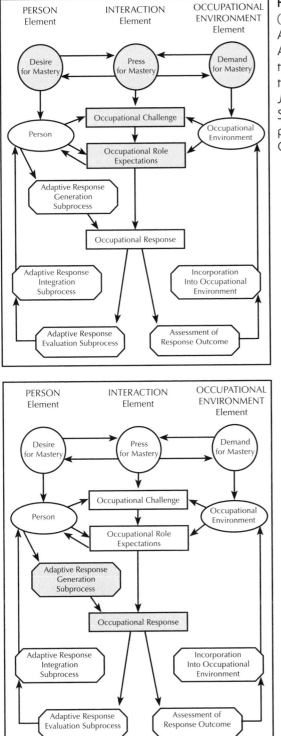

Figure 5-4. Occupational challenge. (Republished with permission of the American Occupational Therapy Association, from Occupational adaptation: Toward a holistic approach to contemporary practice, part 1. *American Journal of Occupational Therapy.* J. K. Schkade & S. Schultz, Vol. 46, 1992; permission conveyed through Copyright Clearance Center, Inc.)

Figure 5-5. Adaptive response generation subprocess. (Republished with permission of the American Occupational Therapy Association, from Occupational adaptation: Toward a holistic approach to contemporary practice, part 1. *American Journal of Occupational Therapy.* J. K. Schkade & S. Schultz, Vol. 46, 1992; permission conveyed through Copyright Clearance Center, Inc.)

Adaptation Energy

"Adaptation energy is the 'fuel' that drives the occupational adaptation process" (Schkade & McClung, 2001, p. 34). Each person or system has a finite amount of energy for the adaptation process and requires conservation so not to exhaust the adaptation mechanism. Two types of adaptation energy exist and include the primary and the secondary. Primary adaptation energy requires intentional effort from the person or system. The use of this adaptation energy quickly exhausts energy resources. Here is an example of primary adaptation energy.

Learning Moment

Think of driving in at night, in a severe thunderstorm for 2 hours. This requires you to pay strict attention to the road. You arrive at your destination, how do you feel and why? Likely you feel tired, worn out, and ready to collapse. This is because you exhausted your energy reservoir.

Primary adaptation energy is appropriately used during the adaptation process at the onset of problem solving. It is not effective, efficient, or satisfying to use primary adaptation energy to continually fuel the process of dealing with an occupational challenge. In doing such, it leaves the person drained, fatigued, and unable to appreciate more creative or complex solutions.

The other type of adaptation energy is secondary. Secondary adaptation energy is the creative energy that fuels adaptation in ways not conceptualized during the use of primary adaptation energy.

The significance of utilizing secondary adaptation energy is that it efficiently and effectively uses the adaptation fuel to solve occupational challenges. Thus, it is not as costly to the energy supply. Using this energy demands less of your energy resources, and your capacity for adaptation and future occupational challenges is greater.

Families who have children with severe autism may experience significant daily behavioral outbursts such as banging their head into the wall, breaking windows, or screaming for hours on end. Families encountering these daily life occurrences rely heavily on their primary adaptation energy to meet their occupational challenges. Here are some examples from research where five families who had a 9-year-old child with severe autism were interviewed (Werner, 2001). The families shared statements such as:

"The whole process (of living) is very difficult...He makes all the basic things a lot harder, whether it is a meal or taking care of everyday activities" (p. 127).

"It's on a daily basis, it's difficult and tiring and stressful and what we might be able to take, what we might be able to handle better in short doses, when it's there day after day after day...it becomes incredible...it's frustrating, and complicates your whole life, your whole family's life is always revolving around this situation" (p. 66).

"It's like having an infant that would have colic...strange behaviors, like self-injurious behaviors... we can take you to walls in our house that have huge holes in it...she just bangs her head...bangs her nose...and goes after her mother and scratches her and hits her. I mean it is an overwhelming path" (p. 86).

From these statements it was apparent the families were overwhelmed and their fuel for adaptation was depleted. The families spent most of their day trying to avoid a crisis. Their adaptation energy was focused on the child with autism, and not on finding ways for the family to engage in effective, efficient, and satisfying occupations. This lifestyle, this way of engaging in occupations, represented families who were trying very hard to make it through their day without an extreme behavioral crisis. The families were depleting their limited supply of adaptation energy. Since the family's frequently instituted solution focused energy as a means for dealing with the demands of having a child with autism, and the units' energy resources were already depleted, the chance for dysadaptive patterns of engaging in occupation was greater.

Learning Activity D

Discuss the following:
1. How can we help individuals shift from using predominately primary adaptation energy to secondary energy?
2. How can we help families shift from using predominately primary adaptation energy to secondary energy?

ADAPTIVE RESPONSE MODES

Adaptive response modes represent the status of the adaptation response mechanism. A person, or a system, can generate a mode of responding that is either an existing adaptation response, a modified form of their previous adaptation response, or a brand new adaptive response. One role of an occupational therapist using OA is to help increase the depth and breadth of a person's adaptation responses. When a person has increased ways of responding adaptively, the likelihood of meeting the demands of current and future occupational challenges is greater.

The development of adaptation responses typically follows a natural course. For example, each of us entered the world with a very limited repertoire of adaptation responses, mainly crying when hungry, wet, or uncomfortable. Within months after birth into this world we developed new ways of adapting to and meeting our occupational challenges. For example, we learned to smile, squeal, or make gurgling noises to obtain a smile from a caregiver. In this process of generating modified and new modes of responding adaptively to occupational challenges our adaptation repertoire was enhanced and expanded.

Initial responses to an occupational challenge typically use existing modes of adaptation. When these modes of adaptation are not effective, efficient, or satisfying to self or society, we alter our strategies for mastering the occupational challenge. Occupational therapy practitioners need to be sensitive to the modes of behaviors the person is exhibiting and pay particular attention to instances where the person attempts to solve each challenge with the same solution.

Learning Activity E

What kind of adaptive response modes are the following children exhibiting and why? What is the role of occupational therapy? Apply these questions to the following scenarios (Figure 5-6):
- Children who abuse drugs and alcohol
- Children who bully others at school
- Children who rock back and forth constantly all day long

Figure 5-6. Detailed view of the adaptive response generation subprocess. (Adapted from Schkade, J., & McClung, M. [2001]. *Occupational adaptation in practice: Concepts and cases.* Thorofare, NJ: SLACK Incorporated.)

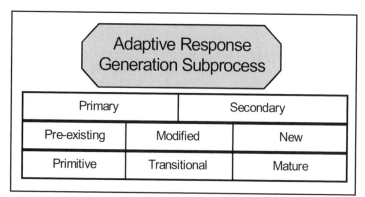

ADAPTIVE RESPONSE BEHAVIORS

Adaptive response behaviors are generated to master and engage in an occupational challenge. By understanding the adaptive response behaviors of a person or system, we gain insight into problem solving and coping responses. Three types of adaptive responses exist and include the primitive (hyperstability), transitional (hypermobility), and mature (exhibiting blended stability and mobility) response behaviors. Adaptive response behaviors occur within and through each person element (e.g., sensorimotor, cognitive, and psychosocial).

Primitive Adaptive Response Behaviors

Primitive adaptive response behaviors are characterized by being stuck or frozen in thought and action. This type of response behaviors is referred to as *hyperstability.* When confronted with an occupational challenge that exceeds a person or systems adaptive capacity, primitive adaptive response behaviors act as a means to restore equilibrium (Schkade & Shultz, 1992). If you have ever felt overwhelmed by an event in your life and unable to conceptualize a plan for action, you were demonstrating primitive adaptive response behaviors. The consequence of being stuck or frozen is the prevention of the generation of new adaptive response behaviors.

Transitional Adaptive Response Behaviors

On the other hand, transitional adaptive response behaviors are characterized by highly variable thought and action. This type of response behavior is commonly referred to as *hypermobility.* When engaging in transitional adaptive response behaviors a person generates a variety of responses, and this increases the likelihood that a solution to the occupational challenge will be generated and used. If you have ever been faced with an occupational challenge, and in the process of trying to solve the challenge you are distracted by numerous events or circumstances in your life, you were demonstrating transitional adaptive response behaviors.

For example, you are sitting down to do your taxes or write a paper and you notice your pencil needs to be sharpened. On the way to getting a new pencil, you remember you had to fold your clothes. However, you pass by the phone and decide to place an order to get a pizza for dinner. In the process of looking up the phone number for the pizza shop you see a coupon for getting your carpets cleaned, and so you look up the number for a carpet cleaner. This is an example of transitional adaptive response behaviors.

Case Vignette #1

I recently supported a family, Ms. Robinson and her two boys, ages 18 months and 2 years. Both children have developmental delays. Her eldest son has severe autism and the younger child is failing to thrive. Upon a visit to her house, she looked withdrawn and sad. When asked what she does during the day, she had a difficult time expressing how she spends her time. Upon observation I watched as she followed the older brother around the house trying to stop him from having a "blow up." She stays at home, except on Fridays when her mother watches the boys so she can go grocery shopping. She told me that she does not have any friends or other means of support. During the day, the younger brother is placed either in his highchair or in a walker. Her adaptive responses behaviors are characterized by frozen thought and actions. She appears overwhelmed and unable to create ways of living that are satisfying, effective, and efficient. Her day tomorrow will look very much like today, and she is demonstrating primitive adaptive response behaviors.

Case Vignette #2

In contrast, consider the family who has a 2-year-old boy with autism and a 5-year-old girl. The family is rarely home and spends their time going to occupational therapy, physical therapy, chelation therapy, play groups, and chiropractic appointments. They have a behaviorist and an occupational therapist come to the home to provide additional therapy. The parents frequently forget when the occupational therapist is visiting the home, even though confirmation phone calls are made. Their home environment is disorganized, with clothing, food, newspapers, and toys covering the living space. When visits do occur, the television is on and the parents "fly" in and out of the room. When asked to describe a typical day, the parents just laugh and say the only thing that is predictable is the unpredictability. The occupational therapist feels the family is "trying very hard" to do the best they can do but they are spending so much time searching for a cure that their lives are chaotic. They are exhibiting transitional adaptive response behaviors.

Mature Adaptive Response Behaviors

When a person or system combines primitive and transition adaptive response behaviors in a "modulated, goal-directed, logical or insightful, and solution-oriented" (Schkade & McClung, 2001, p. 42) manner, mature adaptive response behaviors are demonstrated. In response to an occupational challenge, a mature adaptive response may be to thoughtfully or spontaneously react in a way so the occupational challenge can be resolved. So a mature adaptive response behavior could be exhibited as hyperstability at one point, such as when you are thinking of how to respond to a challenge. Within that same challenge, a hypermobile response may be demonstrated during the process of trying to find a solution. However, the difference between mature and the primitive and transitional adaptive behaviors is the degree to which one loses control of the situation.

For example, your work is hosting a party tomorrow and you were to bring the dessert. You forget about your responsibility until it is 10 at night and remember as you were brushing your teeth and getting ready for bed. You look into the mirror, with toothbrush in hand and think "oh my goodness." You do not move for 2 minutes. Finally an idea to check the pantry comes to you. So you hustle into the kitchen, and open up the pantry and find a few different types of cake mixes. You pull them out and beginning reading the directions and you remember that you do not have any eggs. You think about calling your neighbors, but it is too late and you believe they are already asleep. You think of going in the car to the local grocery store to purchase a dessert, but it is too late and it is closed. Then the idea of getting up early and going to the grocery store in the morning before work to buy a pre-made dessert comes to you. It is a perfect solution, because the grocery store opens at 6 a.m., and you do not need to be at work until 8 a.m. This illustrates the blend of adaptive response behaviors.

Learning Activity F

1. You are working with a 1-year-old child with anencephaly and his family. He has significant motor, hearing, and vision impairment. In fact, he cannot sit, roll, or crawl and responds only to touch. When working with him on understanding his environment, how much time do you allow for him to make an adaptive response? Do you put your hands on him immediately? How does this affect the generation of adaptive response behaviors?

2. What does a person's adaptive response behavior mean for intervention planning? What types of intervention are most suitable for persons demonstrating primitive or transitional adaptive response behaviors?

3. What does a family's collective adaptive response behavior mean for intervention planning? What types of intervention are most suitable for families demonstrating primitive or transitional adaptive response behaviors?

The Adaptation Gestalt

As a person or system generates the adaptation response needed to meet an occupational challenge the response is created through each person element: the psychosocial, sensorimotor, and cognitive. The degree to which each person element is used depends upon the task and person preferences. For example, the adaptation response to learning how to play badminton may require primarily the sensorimotor element. However, following the rules and interacting with the coach will require the involvement of the cognitive and psychosocial elements. "The adaptation gestalt is a straightforward way to conceptualize how an individual 'plans' an occupational response" (Schkade & McClung, 2001, p. 56).

APPLICATION

Research on families with children diagnosed with autism showed families spent a significant portion of their day generating adaptive response behaviors by using their cognitive resources (Werner, 2001). The families constantly contemplated ways to orchestrate family routines around those tolerated by their child with autism. The families planned where they could go out to dinner and knew the child with autism would endure the dining experience. Other times, the family had to coordinate who would stay with the child with autism and for what tasks and when they would switch this responsibility. Additionally, the families had to plan what to take wherever they went so they could deal with any potential problems that may arise with the child with autism. Orchestrating these "complicated" experiences drew upon the family's emotional and cognitive resources. Their energy for adaptation was exhausted from the constant planning which often resulted in feelings of frustration and sadness. This resulted in rigid patterns of daily living, which revolved around those experiences tolerated by the child with autism. The family's use of support networks (social) or sensorimotor preferences were minimal.

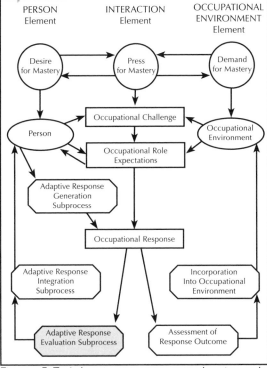

Figure 5-7. Adaptive response evaluation subprocess. (Republished with permission of the American Occupational Therapy Association, from Occupational adaptation: Toward a holistic approach to contemporary practice, part 1. *American Journal of Occupational Therapy.* J. K. Schkade & S. Schultz, Vol. 46, 1992; permission conveyed through Copyright Clearance Center, Inc.)

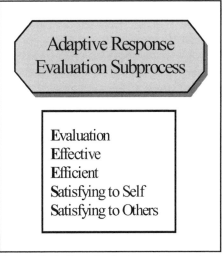

Figure 5-8. Detailed view of the adaptive response evaluation subprocess. (Adapted from Schkade, J., & McClung, M. [2001]. *Occupational adaptation in practice: Concepts and cases.* Thorofare, NJ: SLACK Incorporated.)

Adaptive Response Evaluation Subprocess

Once a person or system has generated and proceeded with a plan in response to the occupational challenge the next step of OA is the evaluation of the outcome. Evaluation of the occupational response is necessary for the internal adaptation process to occur. If evaluation does not occur, the potential for limited growth of the adaptation repertoire is likely. Thus, if a person or family does not have the capacity or the insight to complete an evaluation of the adaptive response, the growth of the adaptation processes will be restricted. Evaluation occurs and is compared against the perceived expectations for mastery. The expectations for relative mastery include the following properties: 1) efficiency of time, energy, and resources; 2) effectiveness, or the extent to which the response achieved the desired goal; and 3) satisfaction to self and society (Figures 5-7 and 5-8).

APPLICATION

In Werner's (2001) research, the occupational challenge was framed as engaging in family occupations. The occupations of these five families focused primarily on the child with autism rather than the unit. Thus an imbalance in their occupational performance occurred as generation of their adaptive response was to the occupational challenge of caring for the child with autism, which placed the occupational challenges of the family unit in an inferior position.

Figure 5-9. Adaptive response integration subprocess. (Republished with permission of the American Occupational Therapy Association, from Occupational adaptation: Toward a holistic approach to contemporary practice, part 1. *American Journal of Occupational Therapy.* J. K. Schkade & S. Schultz, Vol. 46, 1992; permission conveyed through Copyright Clearance Center, Inc.)

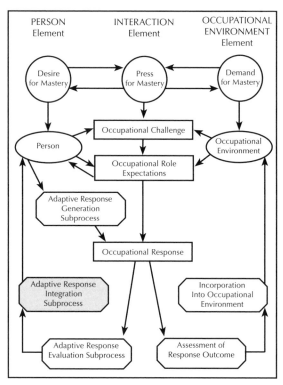

The daily hassles the families felt in caring for the child with autism indicated that the evaluation of their adaptive responses were inefficient, ineffective, and nonsatisfying both to self and society. The families were generally unable to incorporate meaningful family activities (e.g., celebrations, shopping) or to address the needs of a sibling. However, the families developed patterns of adaptation, which averted significant and overt crisis for the family. Thus, the families continued to integrate these ways of adapting into the family element.

The conversations this author had with the families gave them a chance to breathe and to reflect on their daily lives. This process of reflecting included the family in an evaluation of their occupational priorities and previously attempted means for coping with their occupational challenges. According to the OA literature, this process of evaluation is an "empowerment tool" (Schkade & McClung, 2001, p. 65) that can help individuals and families identify which responses are satisfactory and which need to be modified. Evaluation of family life is needed to examine what it would take to generate new patterns of adaptation. Without this, the process may result in the generation of dysadaptive behaviors, which may lead to later occupational regret.

Adaptive Response Integration Subprocess

Following the evaluation of the adaptive response, the person or family takes the information gained during the evaluation and uses it to meet their desires and the environmental demands of future occupational challenges. During the adaptive response integration subprocess is the time when either the adaptive capacity of the individual or system will grow, stay the same, or diminish. One of three states of adaptation results from the integration subprocess and includes OA, homeostasis, or occupational dysadaptation (Figure 5-9).

By integrating the information into the being of the person or the system, the information becomes available for future use in addressing occupational challenges. It demonstrates the degree to which the individual or system has learned about refining the adaptation process and/or searching for new ways of responding adaptively in the future. According to Schkade and McClung (2001), "there are certain indicators that the occupational adaptation process is functioning as the individual confronts and responds to occupational challenges:

1. The client will be experiencing increased relative mastery as he or she responds to occupational challenges.

2. The client will demonstrate spontaneous generalizations to novel tasks without prompting by the therapist or others.

3. The client will initiate adaptations not previously seen or specifically suggested" (p. 71).

Evaluation of the Occupational Environment

In addition to the adaptation processes expressed by a person or family, OA takes into account the demands and expectations of the occupational environment. These include the physical, social, and cultural aspects of the environment. Each of these aspects either support or constrain occupational engagement and thus contribute to the nature of the occupational challenge. After the person or family generates an adaptation response, the environment may or may not evaluate how that person or family engaged in occupation and was affected by the characteristics of the environment. The degree to which the occupational environment evaluates performance depends on the proximity to the person. For example, the occupational environment of the family context may be more responsive to an individual's dysadaptation than a local franchised restaurant. Additionally, when the occupational environment is responsible for the occupational success of the individual there may be more attention given to the aspects of the environment which needs to be modified.

LEARNING MOMENT

In a school setting a child who has attention deficit disorder may have difficulty meeting the expectations of the classroom setting. These expectations include being quiet, finishing classroom work, raising a hand before asking questions, and writing legibly. The student may be constrained by the physical aspects of the environment, such as hearing the teacher's voice clearly or being distracted by visual stimuli. After evaluation of the environment, the teacher may introduce technology to assist with filtering out additional auditory input and place the child at the front of the classroom, away from distractions.

Learning Activity G

In what ways could the social and cultural aspects of the environment contribute to the inability of the student to experience relative mastery in his or her occupational role of being a student (Figure 5-10)?

Figure 5-10. Response of the occupational environment. (Republished with permission of the American Occupational Therapy Association, from Occupational adaptation: Toward a holistic approach to contemporary practice, part 1. *American Journal of Occupational Therapy.* J. K. Schkade & S. Schultz, Vol. 46, 1992; permission conveyed through Copyright Clearance Center, Inc.)

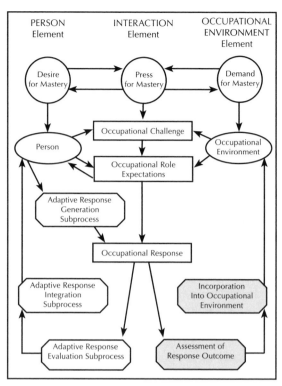

Incorporation Into Occupational Environment

Regardless of proximity, environments can be modified to support occupational performance. To be incorporated into the occupational environment, the environment will need to attach meaning to the outcome of the individual or system experiencing success in occupational engagement. One of the occupational therapist's roles is to help the occupational environment understand the importance of change for current and future occupational performance. Currently one challenge for many occupational therapists practicing in the school setting is helping children with disabilities be in the same settings with their typically developing peers. In this case, we need to bring empirical evidence to show the benefits of inclusion. Additionally, our roles may be to educate the public to modify their values or beliefs about children with disabilities and engagement in occupation.

Summary of Occupational Adaptation as a Model

The process of OA refers to the internal phenomenon that occurs within a person when occupation and adaptation become integrated (Schkade & Schultz, 1992). OA is a state of competency which human beings desire to acquire and a process where a person or family meets an occupational challenge through experience of relative mastery. The process of OA is complex and simultaneously occurs during events in everyday life. The interaction between the person and the environment affords many occupational challenges each day for adaptation. The robustness of adaptation depends upon the capacities and capabilities of the person or family and the responsiveness of the environment to support occupational engagement. Before discussing intervention it will be helpful to review what Schultz and Schkade (1992) developed as assumptions for the model of OA:

1. Occupation provides the means by which human beings adapt to changing needs and conditions, and the desire to participate in occupation is the intrinsic motivational force leading to adaptation (p. 829).

2. OA is a normative process that is most prominent in periods of transition both large and small. The greater the adaptive transitional needs, the greater the importance of the OA process, and the greater the likelihood that the process will be disrupted (pp. 829-830).

3. All three systems are present and active in every occupational response (p. 831).

4. Because of the desire for mastery, the person intends to produce a response to the occupational challenge that will be adaptive and therefore will lead to mastery (p. 833).

5. Adaptation energy is a finite, although adequate, supply of energy present at birth, the bounds of which are idiosyncratic to each person (p. 833).

6. Adaptation energy operates at two levels of awareness (p. 833).

7. It is common for persons to respond to occupational challenges with existing modes whether or not they are appropriate to the task. Only as these modes fail to produce relative mastery outcomes do modified or new modes develop (p. 834).

8. Hypermobile behaviors offer more promise than hyperstable behaviors because they provide variability. This variability may ultimately produce a response that results in a successful outcome (p. 834).

9. Expression of mature behaviors in response to one occupational challenge does not guarantee mature behaviors in subsequent situations. Human beings use all three classes of behaviors as a function of the nature of the challenge, the person's experience with similar challenges, and the difficulty of the challenge as perceived by the person (p. 835).

10. Relative mastery is the extent to which the person experiences the occupational response as efficient (use of time and energy), effective (production of the desired result), and satisfying to self and society, that is, it is pleasing not only to the self but also to relevant others as agents of the occupational environment (p. 835).

11. With evaluation, the occupational event is placed at some point on a continuum from occupational dysadaptation to OA with homeostasis as a midpoint (p. 835).

12. The person's state of occupational functioning is changed as a result of an occupational event. One of three states of occupational functioning is reinforced as a result: OA, homeostasis, or occupational dysadaptation (p. 835).

The Occupational Therapist's Role

OA is about restoration of the adaptation process so engagement and relative mastery in occupation is experienced. The therapist is considered to be a facilitator or enticer, helping the person or family to desire engagement and experience relative mastery with an occupational challenge (Schkade & Schultz, 1992). OA as a model provides a structure for naming and framing the variable nature of a child or the family's occupational performance. It provides a way to understand the occupations of the child or the family, a means to assess the child's or family's adaptive repertoire and evaluate the environmental supports and barriers. It provides an organized way of thinking about the continuum of occupational function and dysfunction. As occupational therapists, we need to discover where the processes of adaptation, evaluation, and integration are disrupting the adaptation process.

We, in collaboration with the person and the context in which the person engages, need to decide who and what will be the focus of our intervention and support.

By framing the intervention with the model of OA, occupational therapists can discern how client factors or contexts are supporting or inhibiting desired outcomes. The model of OA provides a theoretically based means for examining and understanding patterns of performance, contexts, and activity demands. Through the use of the model the following can be identified and assessed: 1) the individual characteristics and desires of the child/family, 2) the environment demands on the child/family, and 3) the ensuing occupational challenge.

— SECTION II —

Assessment

During therapeutic assessment it is particularly important to recognize and document each phase of the OA process. The process includes both person and environmental responses. By gathering this information the occupational therapist will gain an understanding of the person or family he or she is supporting in order to create the most appropriate plan of support and intervention.

The process of assessment begins with interviewing the person or family or primary caregiver to understand the occupational challenge. Table 5-1 outlines the area of the OA process and corresponding questions to elicit information about the occupational challenge and current adaptation responses.

Table 5-2 describes the relationship between the assessment process for OA and the *Occupational Therapy Practice Framework* (AOTA, 2002). Suggested tools for measurement and assessment have been included.

INTERVENTION PLANNING

According to OA, two types of intervention options exist. One of these options frames intervention according to supporting the development of occupation through readiness activities. Occupational readiness activities target specific components of occupational performance dysfunction. For a child who has difficulty with handwriting, one option for an occupational therapist to choose is to improve fine motor strength, coordination, and dexterity. For a child with autism, readiness activities may focus on those critical skills needed to achieve the outcome that frequently involve the areas of communication, social interaction, and emotional regulation.

Interventions that address the core features of why the child and/or family are having difficulty engaging in their desired outcomes are termed occupational activities. With this type of intervention the therapist acts like a coach, helping the client to problem solve through the occupation and critically evaluate his or her performance within the context of occupational performance. Table 5-3 illustrates appropriate intervention activities for the various aspects of adaptation.

Table 5-1

OA ASSESSMENT

Area of the OA Process	Sample Questions for Interview
Understanding the Person	What are some things you/your family/your child has to do? What are some things you/your family/your child wants to do? What are some things you/your family/your child would like to do? What are some things you enjoy doing with your child? What are some things you/your child enjoys? Describe how your child plays or enjoys leisure time. How do you know your child is enjoying this? When does your child seem to do his or her best? How does your child communicate with you? What happens if you don't understand, what does your child do? Describe what your child does alone and with others. How does he or she play/interact with others?
Understanding the Occupational Environment	Walk me through a day in your life/your child's life. What are some rules your family has? Tell me about your parenting styles. Tell me about your classroom rules. What are some barriers you encounter every day? Sometimes encounter? What are some experiences that you know will be challenging to you/your child? Why? Who do you/does your child spend the most time with? Tell me about your/your child's friendships.
Identifying Desired Outcomes	When you think about your/your child's future, what picture do you want to come to mind? What are your hopes and dreams? What are some things your child needs to grow and develop? What are some things your family needs or would find helpful? What are some things that worry you or keep you up at night?
Prioritizing and Measuring Desired Outcomes	At this moment how happy or how satisfied are you with your performance in [*the desired outcome*]? Do you feel effective? Do you feel efficient? If you had to list your goals and prioritize them on a scale from 1 to 10, what would that look like?

continued

Table 5-1 (continued)
OA ASSESSMENT

Area of the OA Process	Sample Questions for Interview
Adaptation Response Energy	As a parent, how do you take time for yourself? Do you feel it is enough to reenergize you? If not, what do you wish you could do to make yourself feel better? How do you find time to relax? What are some things you find relaxing?
Adaptation Response Mode and Adaptation Response Behavior	How does your family usually solve problems?
Adaptive Response Evaluation	How do you feel about your day? What could make your day better?
Adaptive Response Integration	Describe some things that you have tried in the past that you have found to be helpful.

CONCLUSION

In conclusion, OA provides a way of viewing and thinking about how persons and systems meet the challenges of everyday life. By using OA as a model, occupational therapists will gain an understanding of a person's desire for engagement in occupation, the environment's demand for mastery, the occupational challenges the person encounters, and how the person adaptively responds to these challenges. By broadening the focus of occupational therapy assessment and intervention to include the child within a system, such as a family or class setting, we will be identifying the critical elements interfering with occupational engagement and well-being. Through this in-depth analysis of adaptation and focused intervention planning, occupational therapists will support clients in experiencing effective, efficient, and satisfying ways of living.

Table 5-2

OA AND THE *OCCUPATIONAL THERAPY PRACTICE FRAMEWORK*

Occupational Adaptation	*Occupational Therapy Practice Framework*	*Select Tools for Assessment/ Measurement*
Person		
Sensorimotor, Congnitive, and Psychosocial	*Occupational Profile:* • Who is the client? • What is the client's occupational history? *Analysis of Occupational Performance:* • Observe performance in desired occupation • Note effectiveness of performance skills and patterns (client factors) • Interpret assessment to identify facilitators and barriers to performance	• Child Preference Indicator (Moss, 1997) • Routines-Based Interview (McWilliam, 2001) • Children's Assessment of Participation and Enjoyment (King et al., 2004) • Preferences for Activities of Children (King et al., 2004) • Sensory Profile (Dunn, 1999) • Pediatric Evaluation of Disability Inventory (Haley et al., 1992) • School Function Assessment (Coster et al., 1998) • Nursing Child Assessment Satellite Training (Sumner & Spietz, 1994)
Occupational Environment		
Physical, Social, and Cultural	*Occupational Profile:* • What contexts support or inhibit desired outcomes? • What is the client's occupational history? *Analysis of Occupational Performance:* • Observe performance in desired occupation • Note effective performance skills and patterns (context, activity demands) • Interpret assessment to identify facilitators and barriers to performance	• Functional Assessment (O'Neill et al., 1997) • Home Observation and Measurement of the Environment (Caldwell & Bradley, 1984) • Observations • Interviews • Pediatric Evaluation of Disability Inventory (Haley et al., 1992) • School Function Assessment (Coster et al., 1998) • Nursing Child Assessment Satellite Training (Sumner & Spietz, 1994)

continued

Table 5-2 (continued)

OA AND THE *OCCUPATIONAL THERAPY PRACTICE FRAMEWORK*

Occupational Adaptation	Occupational Therapy Practice Framework	Select Tools for Assessment/ Measurement
Occupational Challenge		
Occupational Challenge and Role Expectations	*Occupational Profile:* • Why are they seeking our services? • What occupations and activities are successful or causing problems? • What are the client's priorities and targeted outcomes? *Analysis of Occupational Performance:* • Refine a hypothesis about client's occupational performance strengths and weaknesses • Collaborate with client to create goals that address target outcomes	• Canadian Occupational Performance Measure (Law et al., 2005) • Partnership and Family Quality of Life Survey (Beach Center, 2003) • Choosing Outcomes and Accommodations for Children (Giangreco et al., 1998)
Adaptation Response Subprocesses		
Occupational Response		• Functional Assessment (O'Neill et al., 1997)
Adaptive Response • Generation • Evaluation • Integration	*Occupational Profile:* • What is the client's occupational history?	• Observation of each element of the adaptive response • Interview
Occupational Environment		
Assessment of Response		• Observation and interview
Incorporation Into Occupational Environment		• Observation and interview
Therapist		
Agent of Environment	• Client-centered approach • Therapeutic use of self • Therapeutic use of occupation or activities • Consultation process • Education process	• Measure of Process of Care (King et al., 1995) • Partnership and Family Quality of Life Survey (Beach Center, 2003)

Table 5-3
INTERVENTION IDEAS

Primary Energy	• Engage in activities to encourage relaxation • Engage in activities for redirecting or diverting attention • Help client to find opportunities to embed preferred activities • Discuss with the occupational environment ways to embed preferred activities during the day • Help client to prioritize the occupational challenges • Educate and work with the occupational environment to modify demands or expectations for occupational performance
Pre-existing and Modified Adaptive Response Behaviors	• Engage client in a self-assessment/monitoring of performance in daily activities • Use a social story to help create new or modify pre-existing response behaviors • Modify the environment to elicit modified response behaviors • Reinforce or reward modified response behaviors
Primitive Adaptive Response Behaviors	• Create opportunities for occupation • Work with client and/or the context in which the client engages to identify possibilities • Engage client in activities to broaden adaptation repertoire
Transitional Adaptive Response Behaviors	• Engage client in self-assessment • Work with client and context to assist with establishing predictable, consistent, and structured routines
Adaptive Response Evaluation	• Engage client in self-assessment or self-monitoring, ideas include: Scrapbooking Journaling Storytelling Behavior chart The Alert Program "How Does Your Engine Run?" www.alertprogram.com Behavior chart

Figure 5-11. Picture of Jack.

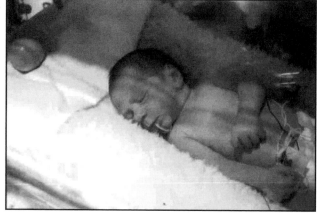

Case Study #1: The Story of Jack and Kim

This story is told by an occupational therapist who describes her time spent with Jack and his mother, Kim.

Jack was born at 27 weeks gestation and Kim at this time was 17 years old. Prior to Jack's birth, Kim was placed on mandatory bed rest at the hospital for 6 weeks and received around-the-clock care and attention. The therapist never heard Kim mention anything about Jack's father.

On the day Jack was born, he entered the world able to breathe on his own and did not require the assistance of a ventilator. Jack was an alert baby and became especially bright eyed and calm when his mother spoke to him. This in turn also affected his physiologic status; his levels of oxygen saturation in his blood would also improve (Figure 5-11).

The therapist had sensed something funny, a red flag, in this first meeting with Kim. The mother talked a lot about religion, and the therapist just knew something did not feel right. Kim said to the therapist that her mother could not come to the hospital and help her with the baby because her mother had experienced a traumatic hospital experience and it was just too hard for her.

The therapist created an opportunity for Kim to create a baby book and journal Jack's journey through the newborn intensive care unit (NICU). Kim was enthusiastic about making the baby book during the first 6 weeks of Jack's life, but then suddenly appeared as if she was not interested. In the beginning, every time she came in she had her nails done, make-up on, and was dressed up. She took many pictures with her baby on these days, posing and wanting multiple pictures taken of her and Jack. Kim never wrote in the journal or in the baby book, but she did like to collect things to put in the book, such as a blood pressure cuff, a label from Jack's bed, and medical equipment used.

As the baby recovered physically, the therapist sensed a second red flag whenever she saw Kim at the baby's bedside, "done-up" in makeup and nice clothes. The mother started flirting with the x-ray technician at the next bed. The therapist felt this is when things began to fall apart with the mother. She stopped coming into the NICU to see Jack and appeared to abandon her baby. The therapists and nurses encourage Kim to come to the NICU by phone, but it does not seem to help. The therapist believes this young mother cannot meet the demands of being a mother, and still has "issues" with her own mother as well.

He was having a typical course in the NICU but had significant reflux, and when a bottle was introduced he had difficulty eating. Jack frequently required all of his feedings to be fed through a tube. The therapist feels Jack had an aversion to stimulation around his mouth. Because he did not eat very well by the bottle, the medical team was discussing the option of placing a permanent feeding tube.

The nurses, doctors, and therapists talked about Kim in unfavorable terms. They described her as not being responsive to authority figures or being told what to do. As Jack's difficulty with taking a bottle continued the staff encouraged Kim to be at as many feedings as possible. He tended to take more liquid through the bottle when his mother fed him, but she rarely showed up for the feedings. The mother took an entire weekend off and did not come to the hospital to feed or visit the baby. The therapist and nurses fed the baby when she was gone, but no real attachment was made with anyone besides the mother. The therapist confronted the mother and said if she wants her baby to go home with her, she needs to demonstrate to the staff that she can feed the baby from a bottle for a few days. Kim does not return to the NICU.

Over the next 2 to 3 months, the baby becomes increasingly withdrawn and the therapist believes "depressed" because his mother is not visiting. On one Friday afternoon, his medical status went from stable and then over the weekend his stomach quit functioning. The nurses and doctors kept him alive as they tried to find his mother. The doctors had to handbag the baby to keep him alive. The mother finally came with other extended family. She stayed at Jack's bedside, but never talked, touched, or tried to soothe him in his pain. The baby died when he was 4 months old.

When the grandmother came to the hospital for the first time in the end, the staff learned that the grandmother is an alcoholic and had abandoned Kim a number of times in her life. This led the therapist to question if the mother had an attachment disorder. Before and after Jack's birth, Kim was homeless and stayed at various people's homes.

Case Study #1 Learning Activity

1. Who is the client?
2. What are the desires of the client?
3. What are the demands of the occupational environment?
4. Describe the occupational challenge.
5. What are the occupational roles of primary concern?
6. Describe the:
   - Client's adaptation energy
   - Adaptive response mode
   - Adaptive response behaviors
   - Experiences of relative mastery
7. If you were the occupational therapist, what types of tools would have been appropriate to understand the client, the environment, and the adaptation process better?
8. What are some ideas for intervention?

Figure 5-12. Picture of Maria by her toy box.

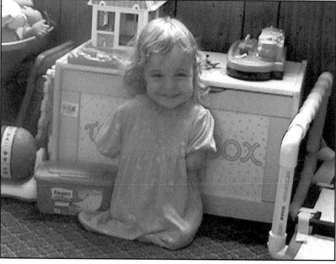

Figure 5-13. Picture of Maria on her ramp.

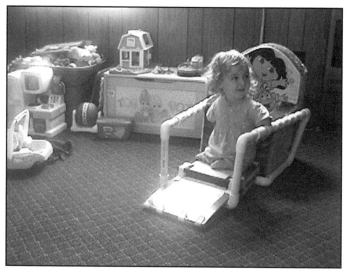

Case Study #2: The Story of Maria, Nita, and Alex

This story is told by an occupational therapist who worked with Maria and her parents, Nita and Alex.

The therapist met the parents through a research study on powered mobility. Maria was the parent's first-born child and she was born without arms or legs. She does have a residual limb on the left upper extremity but it is only a few inches in length. Nita and Alex were in their early 20s when they had Maria, and lived in a rural town on a dirt road in a mobile home. Reportedly they both struggled throughout their schooling.

Nita and Alex's hospital experience after Maria's birth was not a positive experience for them. As word spread around the hospital about Maria, the medical team "paraded" residents, students, and other medical staff through Maria's room to see a child born without arms or legs. Nita and Alex felt that Maria was being treated like a "circus act." The hospital did not provide much hope or preparation before sending them home with their new baby girl. Nita seemed depressed because of not knowing what to expect or hope for Maria's future (Figures 5-12 through 5-14).

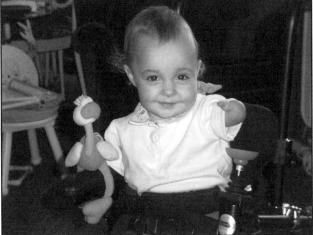

Figure 5-14. Picture of Maria.

An occupational therapist came to provide early intervention services for Maria before she was 6 months old. The therapist tried to adapt or set up the environment to meet Maria's needs. One intervention was a custom seat with supports for Maria to sit upright in when she was 6 months old. Nita took Maria to a local charity hospital and they recommended having prosthetic arms made. However, Nita would get frustrated with the hospital because her child could not do as much with the prosthetic on as she could with it off, but Nita felt the hospital kept pushing her. Nita feel like she was a bad mother because she did not make Maria use her prosthetic arm. Nita did not know how much to push Maria, but the therapists reassured her that it was okay to disagree with something an outsider says because as her mother, she ultimately knows what Maria does best where she lives and plays.

As part of the research study, Maria was provided a power wheelchair when she was 14 months old. Maria had just started sitting up but was not yet shifting her weight laterally. They placed a modified joystick that was higher for Maria to reach with her residual limb, and they worked with Nita to find the best fitting joystick.

Maria used problem solving for activities and learned how to do the activities without adaptations. Maria loved to look at books, using a page puffer, but she eventually wanted the page puffer taken off. She also used her mouth to pick up toys, and then progressed to using her mouth to pick up a toy on the floor and get back up. The therapist placed Velcro rings on all Maria's toys, so she could slip them on her limb and carry them around. Maria could also feed herself with silverware with the shaft bent enough to hang over her residual limb. She did have a difficult time scooping food with a spoon in bowls though. Maria learned to bottom scoot and then progressed to bottom scooting up inclines at around 30 months old. She would practice bottom scooting with three-ring binders and PVC pipe to get to a toy chest or a higher chair. Maria learned to scoot very quickly across the trailer.

The therapist praised Maria for having accomplished so many things and encouraged Nita and Alex to be proud and supportive of Maria's activities. Nita was concerned that Maria did not understand she was different and was worried about what would happen when she did find out she was different. The therapist encouraged Nita and Alex that Maria would be able to do all the same things as the other children her age, but that she would do the activities just a little different. When Maria was 3 years old, Nita finally felt comfortable calling the therapist and was no longer ashamed to seek help.

Maria stayed at her grandmother's house occasionally, but primarily at her mother's house while her mother was not working. When Nita went back to work, she began attending daycare in the 3-year-old program. They wanted to put her in a 4-year-old school program the following year. When the school representatives came to their mobile home, Maria put on a "show," talking and moving about the living room. The school representatives said the only option for Maria would be a classroom for children with developmental disabilities at their school. The speech therapist at the school spoke up and said that program was not appropriate for her and she belonged in the school's 4-year-old program. The school was very apprehensive about letting Maria start and this worried her parents. The occupational therapist reassured the school that she may need slight adaptations in the beginning but, as always, Maria would figure out what works for her to meet those challenges. Maria is thriving in the classroom and has developed many friendships.

Case Study #2 Learning Activity

1. Discuss Maria's adaptation repertoire.
2. How did the occupational therapist facilitate Maria's engagement in occupation?
3. How did the occupational therapist enhance the parents' occupational role?
4. How did the family's capacity for adaptation change over time?
5. How did the occupational environment change?

Acknowledgments

I would like to thank Dr. Toby Hamilton, Dr. Janette Schkade, Dr. Maria Jones, Dr. Laurie Mouradian, Ms. Traci Castles, and Ms. Tera Lindsey for their assistance during the writing of this chapter.

References

American Occupational Therapy Association. (2002). *Occupational therapy practice framework: Domain and process*. Bethesda, MD: Author.

Beach Center on Disability. (2003). *Partnership and Family Quality of Life Survey*. Beach Center, The University of Kansas, KS.

Caldwell, B. M., & Bradley, R. H. (1984). *Home Observation and Measurement of the Environment—Revised*. Little Rock, AR: HOME Inventory, University of Arkansas.

Coster, W., Deeney, T., Haltiwanger, J., & Haley, S. (1998). *School Function Assessment*. San Antonio, TX: The Psychological Corp.

Dunn, W. (1999). Development and validation of the short sensory profile. In W. Dunn (Ed.), *The Sensory Profile Examiner's Manual*. San Antonio, TX: The Psychological Corp.

Garrett, S., & Schkade, J. K. (1995). The occupational adaptation model of professional development as applied to level II fieldwork in occupational therapy. *American Journal of Occupational Therapy, 49*, 119-126.

Giangreco, M. F., Cloninger, C. J., & Iverson, V. S. (1998). *Choosing outcomes and accommodations for children: A guide to educational planning for students with disabilities* (2nd ed.). Baltimore: Paul H. Brookes Publishing Co.

Gibson, J., & Schkade, J. K. (1997). Effects of occupational adaptation treatment with VA. *American Journal of Occupational Therapy, 51,* 523-529.

Haley, S. M., Coster, W. J., Ludlow, L. H., Haltiwanger, M. A., & Andrellos, P. J. (1992). *Pediatric Evaluation of Disability Inventory.* San Antonio, TX: The Psychological Corp.

Hamilton, T. B. (2001). *Occupational adaptation and relationship to narrative in memoirs of adults with acquired disability.* Unpublished doctoral dissertation, Texas Woman's University, Denton, TX.

King, G., Law, M., King, S., Hurley, P., Hanna, S., Kertoy, M., Rosenbaum, P., & Young, N. (2004). *Children's Assessment of Participation and Enjoyment (CAPE) and Preferences for Activities of Children (PAC).* San Antonio, TX: Harcourt Assessment.

King, S., Rosenbaum, P., & King, G. (1995). *The Measure of Process of Care (MPOC): A means to assess family-centered behaviors of health care providers.* Hamilton, Ontario, Canada: Neurodevelopmental Clinical Research Unit, McMaster University and Chedoke-McMaster Divisions of the Hamilton Health Sciences Corp.

Law, M., Baptiste, S., Carswell, A., McColl, M., Polatajko, H., & Pollock, N. (2005). *Canadian Occupational Performance Measure* (4th ed.). Ottawa, Ontario, Canada: CAOT Publications.

McWilliam, R. A. (2001). *Functional intervention planning: The routines-based interview.* Chapel Hill, NC: Frank Porter Graham Child Developmental Center.

Moss, J. (1997). *The Child Preference Indicator.* Center for Interdisciplinary Learning and Leadership, College of Medicine, University of Oklahoma Health Sciences Center.

O'Neill, R. E., Horner, R. H., Albin, R. W., Sprague, J. R., Storey, K., & Newton, J. S. (1997). *Functional assessment and program development for problem behavior: A practical handbook.* Pacific Grove, CA: Brooks/Cole.

Schkade, J. K. (1999). Student to practitioner: The adaptive transition. *Innovations in Occupational Therapy Education, 1,* 147-156.

Schkade, J. K., & McClung, M. (2001). *Occupational adaptation in practice: Concepts and cases.* Thorofare, NJ: SLACK Incorporated.

Schkade, J. K., & Schultz, S. (1992). Occupational adaptation: Toward a holistic approach to contemporary practice, part 1. *American Journal of Occupational Therapy, 46,* 829-837.

Schkade, J. K., & Schultz, S. (2003). Occupational adaptation. In P. Kramer, Hinojosa, & C. B. Royeen (Eds.), *Perspectives in human occupation. Participation in life* (pp. 181-221). Baltimore: Lippincott, Williams & Wilkins.

Schultz, S. (1996). *Treating students with behavior disorders: An institute.* Paper presented at the American Occupational Therapy Conference, Orlando, FL.

Schultz, S. (1997). *Treating students with behavior disorders: An institute.* Paper presented at the American Occupational Therapy Conference, Orlando, FL.

Schultz, S., & Schkade, J. K. (1992). Occupational adaptation: Toward a holistic approach to contemporary practice, part 2. *American Journal of Occupational Therapy, 46,* 917-926.

Schultz, S., & Schkade, J. K. (1994). Home health care: A window of opportunity to synthesize practice. *Home & Community Health, AOTA Special Interest Section Newsletter, 1*(3), 1-4.

Schultz, S. & Schkade, J. K. (1997). Adaptation. In C. Christiansen & C. Baum (Eds.), *Occupational therapy: Enabling function and well-being* (2nd ed., pp. 458-481). Thorofare, NJ: SLACK Incorporated.

Sumner, G., & Spietz, A. (1994). *NCAST Caregiver/Parent-Child Interaction Scales.* Seattle: NCAST Publications, University of Washington, School of Nursing.

Werner, E. A. (2001). Families, children with autism and everyday occupations. *Dissertation Abstracts International, 62*(4), 1835. (UMI No. 3012896).

6

ECOLOGY OF HUMAN PERFORMANCE MODEL

Winnie Dunn, PhD, OTR, FAOTA

Learning Objectives

At the end of this chapter, the reader will be able to:

- Articulate the key features of the Ecology of Human Performance (EHP) model.
- Compare and contrast the EHP model to other models.
- Identify salient factors in a narrative to inform the clinical reasoning process using the EHP model.
- Design an assessment plan that enables a therapist to determine what person, task, and context features are contributing to and interfering with participation.
- Construct an occupation-based intervention plan using the EHP model intervention structure.

— SECTION I —

Overview of the Model

There are many ways to characterize the important factors that enable us to understand the relationships among people, their surroundings, and the activities they choose for their lives. The Ecology of Human Performance (EHP) model was developed by the faculty of the Department of Occupational Therapy Education at the University of Kansas. We, the faculty, designed this model for three purposes originally. First, to create a framework for all the scholarly work that would be produced from our department. Second, the authors wanted to have a means for organizing the curriculum that would communicate our perspectives to students at our university. Third, and most importantly, the authors wanted to create a model that could be used with interdisciplinary colleagues to plan integrated strategies together. The EHP model has been an extremely useful tool to meet all these purposes.

In this chapter we will explore the EHP model and how to use this model as a structure for occupational therapy practice with children, families, and other professionals that serve children.

The EHP model includes the constructs of person, context, task, and performance. When we originally designed the EHP, we emphasized the relationships with context because it has been neglected in both occupational therapy practice and other services as well. For example, comprehensive assessments commonly focus on measuring a child's skills and abilities, but few target the relationship between performance and context. We must consider the relative importance of person skills and abilities and context factors for each particular task performance in comprehensive assessment.

One of the most helpful benefits of including context is that intervention options expand. The EHP offers five intervention approaches: establish/restore, adapt/modify, alter, prevent, and create. The establish/restore intervention addresses changes in the child's skills and abilities (sometimes referred to as remediation). Context and task issues are addressed through the adapt/modify and alter interventions. Prevent and create strategies can focus on the person, context, or task, but are used before a problem occurs or when no problem exists. These intervention options enable professionals to change their emphasis from "fixing" the person to considering a wider range of factors that might be affecting participation in many settings. These intervention approaches are also identified as treatment planning and implementation strategies in the *Occupational Therapy Practice Framework* (American Occupational Therapy Association [AOTA], 2002)

One difference between the EHP and other models lies in the terminology used. The authors did not use the term "occupation" in the model. This decision was made because one of the purposes in creating the model was to collaborate with colleagues from other disciplines. Since the model was not designed exclusively for occupational therapy, the word "task" was used because it is familiar and common in everyday language. The EHP model has been used with interdisciplinary projects. In work with special educators working to support individuals with disabilities in adult education and welfare-to-work programs, the EHP functioned as the theoretical structure for the intervention materials (Bulgren, Gilbert, Hall, Horton, Mellard, & Parker, 1997). Another team developed an environmental assessment for older adults using the EHP as their structure (Teel, Dunn, Jackson, & Duncan, 1997). This is not an attempt to diminish the importance of the construct of occupation in model development. Occupations occur when the person derives meaning from performance of tasks within particular contexts (Christiansen & Baum, 1997, Clark et al., 1991, Nelson, 1996). However, since we sought to create an interdisciplinary structure, other words were chosen (Dunn, Youngstrom, & Brown, 2003).

CORE CONSTRUCTS

There are three core constructs in the EHP model: person, task, and context; the relationship among these constructs enables us to understand a fourth construct, the person's performance. Definitions for each of these four constructs (person, task, context, and performance) are outlined below (Dunn et al., 2003).

Person

Individuals are unique and complex. The person brings experiences; personal interests; and sensorimotor, cognitive, and psychosocial skills, which are referred to as "person variables" in the EHP model. Context can have an affect on the person's interests and either supports or inhibits the person's ability to use his or her skills and abilities (Dunn, Brown, & McGuigan, 1994; Dunn et al., 2003).

Task

In the EHP model, tasks are viewed as objective sets of behavior. When tasks are combined, persons participate in desired occupations to accomplish goals. The demands of a task determine which specific behaviors the person will need to participate successfully. Tasks are universal, vary greatly, and are theoretically available to every person. However, the person's skills, abilities, and interests, combined with participation demands and features of the context, will determine which tasks are used.

Context

Context includes the temporal (including age, life cycle, and expectations related to these aspects), physical, social, and cultural aspects of the environment (Dunn et al., 2003). The EHP model proposes that the interaction between person and context is a critical feature that determines what behaviors and level of participation will be possible. In this way, from the EHP point of view, performance and participation cannot be understood outside of context. Contexts can support or create barriers to participation. For example, persons need certain objects and materials for certain tasks (e.g., books for reading, a comb for hair grooming). Persons also need other people for tasks such as a competitive sport or when learning to play the piano from a teacher. Finally, persons meet with expectations about how to perform within certain contexts (getting to the bus on time, wearing appropriate clothing to a party).

Performance

Persons use their skills and abilities to act within the context. Each person has a performance range, or the number and types of tasks available to the person (Dunn et al., 2003); we can figure out what a person's performance range is by considering the interaction between the person variables (their skills, abilities, and motivations) and the context variables (the supports and barriers).

RELATIONSHIP AMONG THE CONSTRUCTS

A diagram was designed to illustrate the relationship among the EHP constructs. Figure 6-1 illustrates that the person is surrounded by and embedded within the context (Dunn et al., 2003). The interdependent relationship between person and context is dynamic; person and context change continuously. When a person acquires a skill or moves to a new setting, the relationship between person and context has to be reconsidered. We have all experienced children who behave differently in different settings. Some settings will be a good match for a particular child, while another setting may be challenging for that child. In Figure 6-1, the capital "T"s symbolize the myriad of tasks available to everyone. The person within a particular context will interact to determine exactly which tasks will be in the repertoire of that person. For example, the task of shooting baskets exists for everyone. However, a particular child may not be interested in basketball, may not have a hoop or ball available, or may have tried and failed at the activity and rejects it.

Figure 6-2 illustrates how occupations might be characterized within the EHP model. Tasks may overlap into several occupations as illustrated. These occupational patterns would also be unique for each person; for some children the role of sibling would include many tasks, as in the big brother in a family that has a new baby. For other children, the role of sibling might be smaller, as with a college student who has a distant sibling in grade school living at home.

Figures 6-3 through 6-5 illustrate various patterns of the performance range within the EHP model. The megaphone-shaped figure illustrates the person's performance range in each figure. In Figure 6-3 a typical person within the EHP model is illustrated, while in

Figure 6-1. Schema for the EHP framework. Persons are embedded in their contexts. An infinite variety of tasks exists around every person. Performance occurs as a result of the person interacting with context to engage in tasks. (Reprinted with permission from Dunn, W., Brown, C., & McGuigan, A. [1994]. The ecology of human performance: A framework for considering the effect of context. *American Journal of Occupational Therapy, 48*[7], 595-607.)

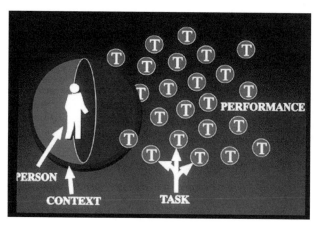

Figure 6-2. Schema of a typical person within the EHP framework. People use their skills and abilities to "look through" the context at the tasks they need or want to do. People derive meaning from this process. Performance range is the configuration of tasks that people execute. (Reprinted with permission from Dunn, W., Brown, C., & McGuigan, A. [1994]. The ecology of human performance: A framework for considering the effect of context. *American Journal of Occupational Therapy, 48*[7], 595-607.)

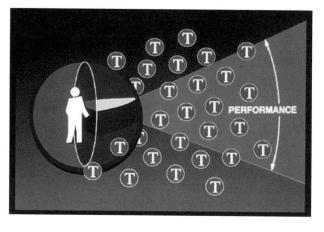

Figure 6-4 a narrower performance range due to the person's skills and abilities being limited is illustrated. In Figure 6-5 a narrower performance range due to a limited context is illustrated. In Figure 6-4 the context is available for performance, but the child does not have the abilities or skills to take full advantage of the context. For example, the child with poor social awareness might not see opportunities that are available to play with peers during free play. In Figure 6-5 the child has the needed skills and abilities, but the contextual resources are not available. For example, an adolescent may know how to drive properly, but may not have a car available.

The final figure, Figure 6-6, illustrates the impact point of the five therapeutic interventions strategies that emerge from the EHP model. Intervention always supports participation, but strategies may be aimed at the person, the context, the task, or in many cases a combination. Let's review the basic parameters of these intervention patterns.

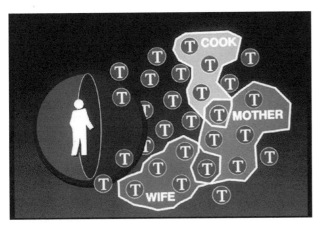

Figure 6-3. Illustration of roles in the EHP framework. Life roles are a constellation of tasks. People have many roles; some tasks fall into more than one role. These role configurations are unique for each person. (Reprinted with permission from Dunn, W., Brown, C., & McGuigan, A. [1994]. The ecology of human performance: A framework for considering the effect of context. *American Journal of Occupational Therapy, 48*[7], 595-607.)

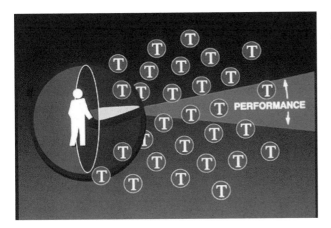

Figure 6-4. Schema of a person with limited skills and abilities within the EHP framework. Although context is still useful, the person has fewer skills and abilities to "look through" context and derive meaning. This limits the person's performance range. (Reprinted with permission from Dunn, W., Brown, C., & McGuigan, A. [1994]. The ecology of human performance: A framework for considering the effect of context. *American Journal of Occupational Therapy, 48*[7], 595-607.)

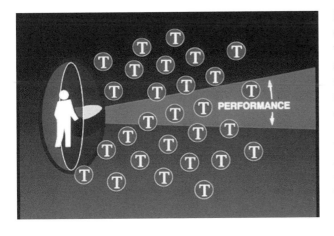

Figure 6-5. Schema of a limited context within the EHP framework. The person has adequate skills and abilities, but the context does not provide the resources needed to perform. In this situation, performance range is limited. (Reprinted with permission from Dunn, W., Brown, C., & McGuigan, A. [1994]. The ecology of human performance: A framework for considering the effect of context. *American Journal of Occupational Therapy, 48*[7], 595-607.)

Figure 6-6. Illustration of thera-peutic interventions within the EHP framework. The arrows indicate the variables that are affected by each intervention. (Reprinted with permission from Dunn, W., Brown, C., & McGuigan, A. [1994]. The ecology of human performance: A framework for considering the effect of context. *American Journal of Occupational Therapy, 48*[7], 595-607.)

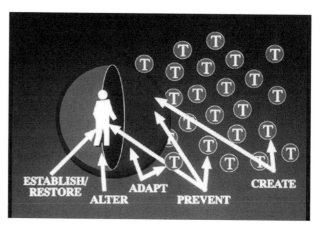

Establish/Restore

The focus of this intervention strategy is the person's skills and abilities. When the child has not had experience in something, the therapist "establishes" the skills. When the child has difficulty or has lost a skill, it is referred to as the "restorative" strategy. Preschoolers may be learning their numbers or taking turns for the first time, and so the occupational therapist's attention would be on collaborating with the teacher to identify ways for the children to establish these skills. An adolescent may need to get endurance back for walking after a rhizotomy, so the therapist would work with the team to restore those previously available skills.

With the primary emphasis on the child's skills, the therapist also weaves in contextual factors as appropriate for the child's outcomes. Perhaps the preschooler needs to have more opportunities for taking turns to get more practice with this new skill. Interventions usually contain more than one of these strategies when placed in the person's actual life routines.

Alter

The focus of this intervention strategy is the context. The practitioner identifies what the child needs to be successful and finds just the right context to support the child to be successful. A therapist might participate with the teachers at a grade level to identify to the teacher the right style to support a particular child's needs. The best match for the child is to be identified, recognizing that contexts contain features that are helpful or interfering for people without any changes occurring. Sometimes just picking the right context can be all that is needed.

Adapt/Modify

The focus of this intervention strategy is on the context or the task. Once we know what the child needs to do, strategies are considered to adjust the demands of the task or change the environmental variables so that the child can be successful. When a parent cuts the tags out of a child's clothing, the parent is making an adaptation so the child can get dressed. When a teacher moves a student to a more remote location in the classroom, he or she is adapting so that the child can get seatwork completed. We make many adap-tations in our lives to make participation easier, more satisfying, or a better fit for our skills.

Prevent

The focus of this intervention is on anticipating problems that might occur and designing strategies to change the outcome prior to the difficulty. Therapists can make educated hypotheses about what might happen when a child has a lot of outbursts in class. Children might begin to avoid this child, creating a problem with social development. Anticipating this, the therapist and teacher might construct small work groups so this child can interact with peers in a more successful way, thus preventing social isolation.

Create

The focus of this intervention strategy is population based. Therapists have a lot of expertise that can be used in many situations other than serving particular disabilities and participation needs of individuals. When we apply this expertise in this larger context, we are providing a "create" intervention. A therapist is providing this type of intervention when serving on the playground development team. The expertise of knowing about movement, development, and motivation, in addition to knowledge about how children with disabilities might access the playground, is a wealth of information for this team. This is an innovative way to employ our knowledge in service to the community's needs.

By including these five intervention strategies, the EHP model provides a window into understanding the complex relationships among person, context, and tasks, creating successful participation. This expansive view of intervention possibilities also enables therapists to understand their comprehensive role in children's lives.

Basic Assumptions of the Ecology of Human Performance Model

As with any model, there are underlying assumptions that form the basis for the model. Underlying assumptions are those ideas and concepts that the authors presume to be true. In the EHP model, the underlying assumptions reflect ideas from many disciplines that are concerned with human behavior and performance. These assumptions were first presented in Dunn, Youngstrom, and Brown (2003), and are summarized here, with an emphasis on children's participation.

THERE IS A DYNAMIC RELATIONSHIP BETWEEN CHILDREN AND THEIR CONTEXTS

1. *It is impossible to understand children without understanding their contexts.* We cannot realize what a child's circumstances, abilities, and expectations are until we are aware of the context for participation. Intervention plans become more relevant as therapists and other team members understand a child's background, friends, classroom arrangement, and demands for performance. When we limit ourselves to scientific knowledge about a child's disability, then the disability begins to define the child's identity. When the team takes a broader look, the disability becomes background, and the participation takes the front seat.

2. *Children and their contexts affect each other.* Children and adults behave differently in different contexts. Two people in the same context derive unique meaning from the context, and so may behave differently. And as soon as a child acts in any way, that action changes the context, and so the child faces a new context in the next moment. The child might have taken a step, thus changing the visual context; or may speak,

thus changing the social interaction demands with others. The teacher moving the desks around will affect the children when they come the next day. Some children will like the change, and others will be skeptical for a while and may be more cautious. Therapists have to keep this dynamic relationship in mind when making recommendations for interventions.

3. *The child's performance range is a function of the child's skills and abilities and the contextual features.* Even when we know a child's disability, we cannot predict what this will mean related to that child's participation challenges. We know that there is a unique experience to understand with each child we serve, and that his or her disability merely provides a background for our overall understanding of the situation. We have the broadest knowledge when we understand what the child can and cannot do, and what the characteristics of the context are that might support or interfere with participation.

CONTRIVED AND NATURAL CONTEXTS ARE DIFFERENT FROM EACH OTHER

1. *We cannot predict whether natural or contrived contexts will elicit the best performance.* Contrived settings have the benefit of being designed for a specific and particular purpose. Children might perform better when contextual variables are controlled in this way. However, children might also have more difficulty in a context that does not have the typical cues needed to interact. For example, a sink in the therapy area might be clean and seem optimal, but it will not contain the soap pump and paper towels the child expects to see for washing his hands. Natural contexts seem messy sometimes. Classrooms are busy and uncontrolled settings; we do not know where noise or movement might come from. Yet, there is a rhythm in the natural context that the child may be relying on to know what to do next. We need to take responsibility for knowing how contexts affect participation before we can see how the best performance can emerge.

2. *A child's true performance will occur in natural environments.* Interdisciplinary evidence is accumulating to indicate that the natural environment is the best place to ensure generalization. Even when an intervention occurs in a contrived setting, therapists have to take responsibility for knowing the impact on participation in the natural environment.

OCCUPATIONAL THERAPY PRACTICE PROMOTES SELF-DETERMINATION AND FULL INCLUSION

1. *Occupational therapy prioritizes what the child wants or needs to do.* This assumption is based on the consumer movement with the person at the center of decision making. For children, we include family and teachers in the process of determining what the child wants and needs to do. The mere fact that everyone is involved in these early decisions increases everyone's motivation to participate in the therapeutic process.

2. *Occupational therapy advocates for children's full rights of participation.* Our profession addresses living the most satisfying life possible. For children this means that we advocate for inclusion in regular education, and that we use our expertise to support children and their teachers so that they can be successful in these school experiences. Occupational therapists can dispel myths, teach alternatives, and create peer supports so that teaching and learning can occur for all the children. When children are older, we support them and their families in finding employment and living situations as well.

INDEPENDENCE OCCURS WHEN WANTS AND NEEDS ARE SATISFIED

1. *Assistive devices support independence, they do not make someone dependent.* Occupational therapists need to view devices as more than supports that encourage dependence. We all use devices to help us throughout the day. Tools in the kitchen, at our desks, and in our bedrooms make tasks easier for us, but they also make it possible for us to get our needs met. The criterion for independence needs to focus on the person being able to direct his or her own life, no matter what devices he or she uses.

2. *Interventions must focus on supporting participation as soon as possible.* From our heritage in the traditional medical model, our profession has had the tendency to prioritize "fixing" problems. When we are taking a broader view, we understand that the priority is to make sure the person can participate as soon as possible. When we adapt a seating arrangement so a child can interact with others, we facilitate social development. This child should not have to participate in a social skills training group first to develop the skills to interact. A team might include both of these strategies in their plans, but it is improper to withhold the contextual and task adaptations that might provide opportunities right away.

Using the Ecology of Human Performance Model in Practice

Any time we use a model in practice, we have the dilemma of explaining it in a stepwise fashion when practice does not actually occur in this way. Practice is fluid and dynamic when serving children, and each insight we have invites us to consider alternatives while keeping our overall outcomes in mind. EHP is a helpful model to apply in practice because it includes intervention strategies that link the practice activities to the conceptual model. The *Occupational Therapy Practice Framework* from AOTA (2002) provides the overall structure for the occupational therapy process. We will use this template to illustrate how the EHP model can be woven in to provide a conceptual basis for practice.

IDENTIFY WHAT THE CHILD WANTS AND NEEDS TO DO

This is a cornerstone of occupational therapy practice. Therapists care about the person's life, so we must begin there. We consult with children, their teachers, their parents, and any other significant individuals in the context.

EVALUATE THE CONTEXTUAL FEATURES

During observations, identify the characteristics of the context that might be supporting or interfering with the child's participation. Consider the physical context, how other people might affect the child, what expectations are present, and what cultural factors might affect the desired performance.

IDENTIFY THE CHILD'S PERFORMANCE FEATURES

Determine both the typical performance and the specific characteristics of the target child's performance so we can begin to formulate what might be interfering with successful participation. Therapists also find out from key stakeholders (parents, child, teacher) what successful performance would look like. Some people will be satisfied with average performance or with an adapted version of performance.

Table 6-1		
PARENTS' PRIORITIES		
Identify What the Child Wants and Needs to Do		
Areas of Occupational Performance	**Occupational Performance Issues**	**Priorities Rated in Order of Importance**
Activities of Daily Living		2
Work/Productivity		1
Play/Leisure		3

ANALYZE THE CHARACTERISTICS OF THE DESIRED TASKS

Occupational therapists then want to consider the task demands, skill requirements, and supports needed for someone to accomplish the desired tasks. We observe and interview people to understand what is necessary for success; this information will enable us to design alternatives and make reasonable recommendations within the contexts of interest.

DEVELOP CONCEPTUALLY BASED HYPOTHESES AND ASSOCIATED INTERVENTIONS

Using the information gathered, begin to formulate ideas about what might be interfering with participation. We ground our ideas in models like the EHP and other practice frameworks so that when we evaluate the effectiveness of our interventions, we can generate alternative interventions if our hypotheses were inaccurate. We do not have to be right every time. Therapists just have to be systematic and grounded in our thinking so that we can make adjustments if children are not making expected progress.

Case Studies Illustrating the Application of the Ecology of Human Performance Model in Pediatric Practice

The case studies that follow use this process to illustrate how the EHP model may be applied in pediatric practice. Readers are invited to work through these case studies with worksheets and questions to guide your thinking, so you can learn how to use the EHP model yourself. Tables 6-1 through 6-5 are blank samples of the worksheets used to work through the case studies.

Table 6-2
CONTEXT DATA WORKSHEET

Name:

Evaluate the Contextual Features

	Code*
Physical	
Social	
Cultural	
Temporal	

*Code: c=contributing factor; b=barrier to performance; ?=could be either

Table 6-3
DATA SUMMARY WORKSHEET

Name:

Tasks:

Identify the Child's Performance Features

Person Variables	Activities of Daily Living	Work/Productive Activity	Play/Leisure
Sensorimotor			
Cognitive			
Psychosocial			

Table 6-4
SUMMARY OF TASK ANALYSIS WORKSHEET

Name:

Analyze the Characteristics of the Desired Tasks

Typical Performance of Task:	Performance

Table 6-5
WORKSHEET FOR OUTLINING THERAPEUTIC INTERVENTIONS

Develop Conceptually Based Hypotheses and Associated Interventions

Performance	Establish/Restore	Alter
Adapt/Modify	Prevent	Create

Case Study #1: Peter

Desire: To participate in work groups successfully at school and ride the bus.

Peter is a 12-year-old sixth grader. He is about to transition into the middle school in his neighborhood. Everyone knows Peter in his elementary school, and the neighborhood accepts his "quirky" behaviors as part of who he is. Peter and his parents are worried about the bigger middle school because there will be many more students and many who don't know Peter. They don't see that they will have opportunities to make sure people feel endeared by Peter's behaviors, and see that this is how he has made it so far. He will just be in the crowd, and they fear that his quirky behaviors will turn into liabilities in this new school. Table 6-6 summarizes Peter's and his parents' priorities as he enters this new school; this forms the basis for assessment and planning

Table 6-6

PETER AND HIS PARENTS' PRIORITIES

Identify What the Child Wants and Needs to Do

Areas of Occupational Performance	Occupational Performance Issues	Priorities Rated in Order of Importance
Activities of Daily Living	Ride the bus to school.	2
Work/Productivity	Participate successfully in work groups at school.	1
Play/Leisure	Having friends in his new school.	3

Case Study #1 Learning Activity A

Identify what the child wants and needs to do.

The occupational therapist decides to analyze the current school setting to get some insights for planning. Table 6-7 provides the contextual assessment of his elementary school. The therapist found potentially helpful and interfering factors that might be important to know as Peter transitions to middle school. She also goes to the middle school and makes a list of possible positive and challenging features there as well. This information will form the basis of forward planning with Peter.

Case Study #1 Learning Activity B

Evaluate the contextual features in this particular case.

The elementary team meets to discuss Peter's abilities and needs as related to his desire to participate in work groups. Prior to the meeting, the therapist has observed Peter to see how he manages in several activities (Table 6-8).

Case Study #1 Learning Activity C

Identify the child's performance features.

Table 6-7
CONTEXT DATA WORKSHEET

Name: Peter

Evaluate the Contextual Features

	Code*
Physical • Peter attends a neighborhood elementary school. • His home is situated in a block with long-standing families who know him well. • He attended the only elementary school in his community, a school with 12 classrooms from kindergarten through fifth grade.	c ? c
Social • Everyone at school (janitor to secretaries) knows Peter. • Peter's mother works part-time to help with Peter's after school activities. • Peter wants to have good work groups. • Peter has one 16-year-old brother, who vacillates about having a brother who "is weird."	c ? c ?
Cultural • Peter's neighborhood is very tightly knit. • The community values athletic and leadership skills. • Peter's grandparents live out of state and keep in touch by email.	? b ?
Temporal • Peter is 12 years old. • Peter has a chronic condition that interferes with communication and behavior (Asperger's syndrome). • He is an elementary student who succeeded in his familiar school and classroom.	? b ?

*Code: c=contributing factor; b=barrier to performance; ?=could be either

Table 6-9 summarizes the impressions about Peter's performance. The therapist also analyzes the characteristics of a work group with the help of the middle school special education teacher.

Case Study #1 Learning Activity D

Analyze the characteristics of the desired tasks.

Table 6-8

DATA SUMMARY WORKSHEET

Name: Peter
Tasks: Daily routines

Identify the Child's Performance Features

Person Variables	Activities of Daily Living	Work/Productive Activity	Play/Leisure
Sensorimotor	Peter gets dressed with familiar music playing in the background.	Peter does chores while it is quiet at home and gets his homework done.	Peter has trouble with noise in large group free play situations.
Cognitive	Peter wants his daily routines to be just right.	Peter needs order; this can help but also can be a problem in the classroom. He perseverates on most tasks.	Peter has trouble initiating and terminating activities; he has trouble with joke telling and after school activities.
Psychosocial	Peter wants to wear "cool" clothes, and sometimes perseverates on particular items as critical.	Peter does not know how to use social skills with work groups.	Peter does not understand facial expressions and misses nonverbal cues, so peer conversations are lost on him.

Table 6-9

SUMMARY OF TASK ANALYSIS WORKSHEET

Name: Peter

Analyze the Characteristics of the Desired Tasks

Typical Performance of Task: Riding the Bus	Peter's Performance
Get on the bus Find a seat quickly Negotiate where to sit Greet other riders Socialize during the ride Take turns when exiting the bus Screen out sounds of traffic, children, bus Stay balanced in seat during ride	Gets on and off bus efficiently Greets others but is lost after that Becomes overwhelmed with the noises and gets agitated Need to find out how he handles the movement of the bus

Table 6-10
WORKSHEET FOR OUTLINING THERAPEUTIC INTERVENTIONS

Develop Conceptually Based Hypotheses and Associated Interventions

Performance	Establish/Restore	Alter
Peter wants to ride the bus.	Peter and his parents will ride the bus during the summer. Neighborhood friends will also ride the bus.	Parents will bring Peter to school on days with special events.
Peter needs to participate in small work groups.	Write a social story about work group participation with Peter.	Peter will join the baseball card club. Peter's work group can go to the library to work.

Adapt/Modify	Prevent	Create
Peter will wear foam earplugs on his MP3 player on the bus ride. Peter will sit in the front of the bus.	Peter will have lunch with the bus driver so that he knows this person.	Not applicable.
Teacher will preassign the duties of the work group.	Provide post-its on the notebook schedule to prevent Peter from becoming agitated about an upcoming work group.	Not applicable.

The therapist would use all of this information and other data from evaluations to generate a number of possible intervention strategies to offer at the team meeting. An example of a list a therapist might generate is provided in Table 6-10.

Case Study #1 Learning Activity E

Develop conceptually based hypotheses and associated interventions.

The district has a transition team that includes professionals from elementary and middle schools and Peter's parents. Peter will participate in a beginning-of-the-year meeting later. Peter's team includes his teachers, principal, occupational therapist, parents, and a special educator. The classroom teacher describes her class as very structured and says that this is useful for Peter. The parents like the visual schedule posted in the room because it keeps Peter on track. (This is an **adaptive** strategy; the teacher keeps students with her and does not wait for a student to get off the schedule). They started doing this because Peter was always interrupting class to ask what was next. This behavior created negative feelings with peers, and so they did not want to work with him on projects. The special educator cautions that changes in the schedule can be tricky because Peter is so inflexible. The middle school principal says that this will be less a problem in middle school, since all class time is so precious to the teachers. He suggests that they make Peter a notebook-sized visual schedule and plan to give Peter a notice when the schedule will be different, with post-its on the visual schedule (also an **adaptive** strategy). The parents are delighted with this advanced planning.

The occupational therapist reported that Peter fidgets and seems to be distracted by movement and noise. The team thinks that they will suggest to his middle school teachers that they place Peter's desk right at the back wall, farthest from the door, to keep students from bumping into him in class (**altering** the context by using spaces and configurations already available). This may reduce his distractibility related to students moving in and out, but Peter can still face the teacher.

The middle school principal says that Peter might want to participate in their accelerated math program. The parents are delighted because Peter loves math. The principal suggests that Peter tutor for math, as a way for students to view him positively right away (**prevention** intervention). They will explore this option when he arrives.

Peter also wants to ride the bus in middle school, but the noise and motion on the bus have always been a barrier. His parents are nervous. The occupational therapist suggests that there are some parts of the bus ride that may be positive for Peter. The vibration might be calming, and if Peter can use something to dampen the noise (e.g., using concert ear-plugs, sitting at the front, using an MP3 player on the bus; **adaptive** and **alternative** strategies). The principal agrees to look into getting Peter on the bus last to reduce his time there. The parents agree to a trial period of sending him to school on the school bus.

Peter is an avid baseball card collector and trader. The middle school has a club with this interest, so Peter can start with this as a work group. Since Peter's memory for sports statistics is large, the team feels this will be a way to get one successful workgroup started (**prevention**).

It is important to note that some of the prevention interventions were adaptive or restorative in the last school. Previously, Peter was having difficulty, which is what led the previous team to design and implement the strategies; this is what made the interventions "adaptive" or "restorative." Now that he is at his new school, the new team can start out with strategies in place to keep his difficulties from occurring, so now those strategies are preventative in nature. **It is the purpose or goal behind the strategy that enables you to determine which EHP intervention you are using.** The EHP interventions provide you with a framework for thinking systematically about your intervention planning. As you can see in Peter's story, the same activity could be classified different ways depending on how you think about it in the child's life.

Case Study #1 Learning Activity F

What if Peter was 18 years old? The team would be looking at community options, including community college, work, and living possibilities. Go through this same process with your classmates and design some plans for Peter with this change in the story. Discuss what Peter will want to do in these new settings, what the characteristics of tasks are, what Peter is doing, and how the contexts might help or create barriers for him. Then, develop some conceptually based hypotheses and recommendations for Peter. Remember, he is old enough in this new scenario to participate in the planning, and he will likely have insights about what will or will not work for him.

Table 6-11
VERONICA AND HER PARENTS' PRIORITIES

Identify What the Child Wants and Needs to Do

Areas of Occupational Performance	Occupational Performance Issues	Priorities Rated in Order of Importance
Activities of Daily Living	We want Veronica to take a more active part in getting dressed.	2
Work/Productivity		
Play/Leisure	We want Veronica to move around more to play.	1

Case Study #2: Veronica

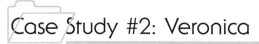

Need: To move around to play.

Veronica is 2.5 years old, who is part of the early intervention services in her county. Her family identified her through the Parents as Teachers program in their state. Veronica is the youngest of four children, and the only girl in the family. She is also the only granddaughter for her grandparents. The parents admit that Veronica is the "princess" of the family. She has been showered with gifts, clothing, and toys for a girl since the family had all boys until Veronica was born. At this point, the Parents as Teachers visitor talked to the parents about the fact that Veronica should be moving around to play and get the things she wants. They decide to get the early intervention providers involved so they could get the ball rolling before Veronica turns 3 and would be eligible for preschool programs. Table 6-11 provides a summary of the family's priorities for Veronica.

Case Study #2 Learning Activity G

Identify what the child wants and needs to do.

Table 6-12 provides a summary of the contextual assessment within Veronica's home.

Case Study #2 Learning Activity H

Evaluate the contextual features.

The occupational therapist visited the home to meet Veronica and her family and gathered initial information the team would need for planning. Since the top priority was Veronica moving around more in play, the therapist also completed an analysis on Veronica's performance skills during play (Table 6-13).

Table 6-12
CONTEXT DATA WORKSHEET

Name: Veronica

Evaluate the Contextual Features

	Code*
Physical • Brothers bring her toys whenever she wants them. • Play areas are in priority places in the family living spaces.	b c
Social • Brothers are very attentive to Veronica during play time. • Mother places Veronica on floor near preferred toys.	? b
Cultural • The family is very child oriented. • The family includes children in most activities and across ages.	c c
Temporal • There are age-appropriate toys around the home. • There are peer models for playing in her brothers. • Veronica's play patterns are like younger children's play patterns.	c c b

*Code: c=contributing factor; b=barrier to performance; ?=could be either

Table 6-13
DATA SUMMARY WORKSHEET

Name: Veronica
Task: Playing

Identify the Child's Performance Features

Person Variables	Activities of Daily Living	Work/ Productive Activity	Play/Leisure
Sensorimotor			Fussy when moved away from vertical positions. Neutral to positive responses to being touched. Noise from brothers seems fine for Veronica. Veronica notices when people enter and exit.
Cognitive			Indicates her needs through gestures and vocalization. Plays with toys like a younger child would. Play is in one- and two-step patterns and repeats.
Psychosocial			Veronica smiles and gives eye contact to everyone in the room. Veronica shares with her brothers. Veronica is pleasant, and nothing seems to bother her.

Table 6-14
SUMMARY OF TASK ANALYSIS WORKSHEET

Name: Veronica

Analyze the Characteristics of the Desired Tasks

Typical Performance of Task: Playing	Veronica's Performance
Changes in planes of activity during play Moving by walking or crawling to obtain toys Experimenting with climbing More active than sedentary toys Some interactive play	Remains in sitting position during play Primarily uses manipulation to play Has some toy preferences Uses toys in a limited way and repetitively Interacts socially during play, but does not interact with toys and movement and other children

Case Study #2 Learning Activity I

Identify the child's performance features.

To identify what might help the planning, the therapist also conducted an analysis of both Veronica's play patterns and what would be expected of same-age peers (Table 6-14).

Case Study #2 Learning Activity J

Analyze the characteristics of the desired tasks.

Using all of this information, the therapist drafted some ideas to present to the family at her next visit (Table 6-15).

Case Study #2 Learning Activity K

Develop conceptually based hypotheses and associated interventions.

When the therapist got to the family's home, they welcomed her to join them. Veronica and two of her brothers were home with mom, while dad and the older brother were at work and school, respectively. The children were playing in the living room; mom and the therapist joined them. Veronica was a happy child and seemed content sitting in the middle of the room. The boys were very attentive to Veronica and seemed to anticipate her every need, bringing toys and taking them away, and talking to her about what to do with the items. Occasionally Veronica would point and vocalize regarding something she wanted and the boys were happy to oblige. When the therapist began interacting with Veronica and offering her toys, one of the brothers offered commentary: "She doesn't really like that toy" and "You have to give her the green part first." Mom got the boys a

Table 6-15

WORKSHEET FOR OUTLINING THERAPEUTIC INTERVENTIONS

Develop Conceptually Based Hypotheses and Associated Interventions

Performance	Establish/Restore	Alter
Veronica needs to move around to play.	Introduce propping, all fours, or standing next to a play surface to encourage new "stability" positions to increase strength, balance, muscle tone, and postural control. Encourage parents to participate in the planning board of the preschool so they can learn what is developmentally appropriate to expect of Veronica.	Enroll Veronica in a Mother's Day Out program to introduce a more diverse social context for play.
Adapt/Modify	**Prevent**	**Create**
Move the toys out of Veronica's reach. Coach the brothers about where to put toys for her. Teach parents and grandparents how to adjust play situations to invite Veronica to move.	Invite neighborhood children to come over and play to prevent Veronica from withdrawing from peers as her skills become more distant from peers.	Encourage parents to participate in the planning board of the preschool so they can contribute a wider perspective to the offerings at the preschool.

snack, so she and the therapist could focus on Veronica. The therapist asked mom to sit out of reach of her daughter and offer her a preferred toy. Veronica was engaging with mom, but made no attempts to move toward the toy. The therapist had mom put Veronica on her tummy and Veronica got a little fussy.

By the end of this visit, the therapist had some hypotheses about the situation. Veronica was definitely below movement and exploration expectations when compared to peers, and this could interfere with her ability to interact when she starts preschool. The therapist was not sure which factors were primary and which factors were contributing to her lack of moving to play. Using the EHP model, she considered all the central concepts. From a "person variable" point of view, it is possible that Veronica had poor postural control, low muscle tone, poor body awareness, or difficulty with motor planning. She could also have some difficulty with sensory processing; for example, if she had low sensory thresholds for vestibular input, this could have led to Veronica keeping her body in one plane related to gravity (thus restricting movement that activates the vestibular organ and creates more input).

Table 6-16

GENERATING HYPOTHESES ABOUT VERONICA'S PLAY

Possible Hypothesis About Why Veronica Is Not Moving to Play	Data Supporting This Hypothesis	Intervention Approach Consistent with This Hypothesis
She is not strong enough (person factors).	She remains stable in sitting during play. She collapses when placed in new positions.	Increasingly incorporate more weight-bearing (tall kneeling, propping), pushing, and pulling.
She is avoiding vestibular input (person factors).	She is fussy when placed in a prone position. She remains stable in sitting which limits vestibular input.	Add variety in carrying routines. Incorporate propped positions for play.
The boys' play is too complex for her to join in (task factors).	The boys roughhouse; she watches them but does not attempt to join them or mimic their movements.	Teach family some games that she can participate in successfully.
The context does not require her to move (context factors).	Mom places her amidst her toys. Brothers bring her any toy she might want. Everyone comes to her in the family room.	Teach family how to invite her to leave her sitting position to get toys and to interact.

From a "task variable" point of view, perhaps the movement activities presented to her via her older brothers may have been too difficult for Veronica, leading to her selecting a more passive observer role. When considering "context variables," it seemed clear that the family was very tuned into Veronica's needs and created an environment in which there were very little demands to move. In their attempts to care for her, entertain her, and please her, they may be supporting her to remain in an immobile position by not pressing her to engage in movement.

The therapist decided to conduct some additional assessments and consult with the physical therapist. The therapists watched a video together (which the occupational therapist made during the home visit) and discuss possible options for why Veronica is not moving and what might be good strategies to get her to move. The occupational therapist also sent home an Infant Toddler Sensory Profile to get some additional information on Veronica's responses during everyday life.

Based on this additional input, the occupational therapist forms some initial hypotheses that she will test during the first several visits with the family. She will also explore with the family which intervention ideas seem the best match for their lifestyle. Table 6-16 provides a summary of the occupational therapist's thinking.

When the occupational therapist met with the family, everyone was there including dad and grandparents. They were all excited to have ideas to help Veronica. Mom was reluctant to discuss some of the issues at first, commenting several times about Veronica being her baby. Grandma and dad broke through the emotional situation and said they saw that they were coddling Veronica and didn't want this to cause a problem for her at school in the future. When they discussed possible reasons why she didn't move, the family was eager to learn strategies to encourage movement during play, and dad said "Maybe she will get stronger if we make her move." So with the boys' help, the occupational therapist directing, and Veronica as the star, they commenced to make a videotape of ways to play with Veronica. All the family got into the act, and the boys loved being operatives. The therapist explained that this way they could keep checking back to see that they were doing the best things for Veronica.

When they talked about the preschool and sitting on the school board, dad thought he would enjoy doing this. Mom said she might do better to visit the school and observe, and thought maybe she could volunteer or work part-time there. They did not like the Mother's Day Out idea because it was held in a church other than their own, which would require all new relationships. They did agree to take advantage of neighborhood connections to find some playmates for Veronica (other than her brothers).

It took the occupational therapist eight visits to get everything in place with the family. After that, she called every 2 to 4 weeks, and then assisted in placement and transition to preschool after Veronica turned 3 years of age.

Case Study #2 Learning Activity L

What if Veronica was an only child of a single parent on welfare? What would change about your data-gathering strategies and the intervention options you might offer the mother? Go through this same process with your classmates and design some plans for Veronica and her mother with this change in the story. Discuss what this mother might want for Veronica, what the characteristics of tasks are, what Veronica's play might look like, and how the contexts might help or create barriers for her. Then develop some conceptually based hypotheses and recommendations for Veronica's mother that are respectful of her family situation.

Case Study #3: Charles

Desire: To be part of the school play.

Charles is a 16-year-old youth who attends the neighborhood high school. He has been finding his way through middle school, and now high school, trying to "get in" with a group of friends. Charles is from an Asian family that is very proud of their heritage and traditions. The family spends a lot of time together and takes an interest in each other's lives. This creates a strong base for Charles, but now that he is in high school he wants to broaden his social network to include peers more. He has been successful getting his parents to include friends in their family events, but now he wants to spend time in their contexts (i.e., with their families and at extracurricular activities). Many of his friends are involved in music and drama, so he has decided he wants to be part of the next play production.

The occupational therapist at Charles's school is a member of the enrichment team. This team of professionals and student members identify and establish a wide range of extracurricular activities for all students so everyone can find something that interests him or her, and can develop strong peer relationships based on common interests. The occupational therapist joined the team as a **create** intervention strategy for the high school. She had been following students from middle school to high school, observing social isolation

	Table 6-17	

CHARLES'S PRIORITIES

Identify What the Person Wants and Needs to Do

Areas of Occupational Performance	Occupational Performance Issues	Priorities Rated in Order of Importance
Activities of Daily Living		
Work/Productivity		
Play/Leisure	I want to be part of the school play so I can spend more time with my friends.	1

and confusion about how to navigate the broader landscape of adolescence. She decided that working at a systems level to get options in place for all students would ultimately be a service both to her students at risk and to other students who were not in special education services but were also struggling to establish their emerging identity. With her psychosocial background, she became a valued member of this team.

It was in this context that Charles and the occupational therapist met. The enrichment team made themselves available to any students who wished to explore options for themselves, but couldn't identify what would be best suited for them. In this interview, the occupational therapist found out that Charles had a solid set of friends and that they were the "artsy" kids at school. Charles said that his issues were that he didn't know whether he wanted to be an actor or dancer in the musical, and that he wasn't so interested in the orchestra. He said that he loved the manual arts classes he had taken, but didn't see any clubs for kids who liked to build. He also told the occupational therapist that he was having trouble with his parents letting him participate in extracurricular activities. Table 6-17 provides a summary of Charles's priorities for his high school experiences.

Case Study #3 Learning Activity M

Identify what the person wants and needs to do.

When the occupational therapist suggested looking into being part of the set crew, Charles was very excited. He asked for help convincing his parents this was a good experience for him.

The occupational therapist finds Charles's family at Welcome Back to School night and introduces herself as a member of the enrichment team. With Charles's permission, she says that she is excited about a contribution that Charles can make to the school this year, and asks when they can meet to discuss it. They agree to meet the next week. The occupational therapist and Charles then set out to create a strong plan, with documentation of the rationale; Charles indicated this would be important for his father particularly. Table 6-18 provides a summary of the contextual assessment related to Charles's participation.

Table 6-18

CONTEXT DATA WORKSHEET

Name: Charles

Evaluate the Contextual Features

	Code*
Physical • The staging area for the plays has a lot of room for building and painting, including supplies and equipment. • The theater stage is large, providing a prominent space for crew handiwork to be displayed.	c c
Social • Many of the "artsy" students participate in the school play. • Charles's friends will be active in the play. • The play director has had Charles in class, so they know each other.	c c c
Cultural • Charles's family is very family oriented (i.e., socializing is within the family). • Charles's family places a high value on productivity and hard work. • Charles's family sees service to those around you as an important characteristic.	? ? c
Temporal • Charles is in a social interaction period of his development. • Charles wants to expand his sense of community and "family."	? c

*Code: c=contributing factor; b=barrier to performance; ?=could be either

Case Study #3 Learning Activity N

Evaluate the contextual features.

Before they met, the occupational therapist also summarized with Charles what skills he would be bringing to the task so they could present a strong argument to his parents (Table 6-19).

Case Study #3 Learning Activity O

Identify the person's performance features.

Table 6-19
DATA SUMMARY WORKSHEET

Name: Charles
Task: Being a member of the set crew for the play

Identify the Person's Performance Features

Person Variables	Activities of Daily Living	Work/Productive Activity	Play/Leisure
Sensorimotor		Manual dexterity and knowledge of how to use tools.	Enjoys interacting with various media required to build the sets.
Cognitive		Perceptual skills about how to put things together. Ability to solve building challenges as they arise.	Generates creative ideas about set design. Understands topographical and spatial relationships.
Psychosocial		Team oriented in his work planning, involves others in decision making and problem solving.	Has a solid set of friends. Interested in developing friendships.

The occupational therapist also interviewed the play director to find out what the expectations would be for Charles's new activity (Table 6-20).

Case Study #3 Learning Activity P

Analyze the characteristics of the desired tasks.

Using all of this information, the occupational therapist and Charles and the play director drafted some ideas to present to the family at the meeting (Table 6-21).

Case Study #3 Learning Activity Q

Develop conceptually based hypotheses and associated interventions.

Table 6-20
Summary of Task Analysis Worksheet

Name: Charles
Analyze the Characteristics of the Desired Tasks

Typical Performance of Task: Building Sets	Charles's Performance
Strength to move planks and backdrops as they are being assembled	Understands physical demands and has basic construction skills from helping dad build a room on house
Team interaction skills to solve construction problems	Exercises regularly so has strength and endurance for lifting, moving
Organization to get set arranged for ease of use during the play	Negotiating skills with peers (served as a peer mediator)
Motivation to keep at the work when it is tedious or takes longer than expected	Efficient with homework and other chores and responsibilities
Building and construction skills or willingness to learn	Teachers say he can be counted on to follow through
Good time management	

Table 6-21
Worksheet for Outlining Therapeutic Interventions

Develop Conceptually Based Hypotheses and Associated Interventions

Performance	Establish/Restore	Alter
Charles wants to be part of the school play.	Help Charles develop a rationale and presentation plan for his parents.	Invite parents to include the play and set areas as extended "family space" by having them come by the school whenever they wish.

Adapt/Modify	Prevent	Create
Design a "family" sitting area for performance night so Charles's family members are seated together.	Support Charles to present to his parents to prevent his resentment and sense of social isolation from not being able to be part of the school activities.	Design extracurricular options for students so all ranges of interests and abilities will have ways to participate in the school.

At the meeting, Charles presented his information based on the analysis and plans that he had worked on with the occupational therapist. He knew this systematic approach would be his best shot with his parents, who liked to make logical decisions. The occupational therapist and play director served as resources.

The occupational therapist provided an introduction to the meeting to frame the discussion. She stated that high school was a place to prepare young people for adult life and described the various roles that would be expected of adults. She said that the school personnel wanted each student to find ways to not only learn what was required in courses, but to also explore their other strengths that might lead to work options or that might be talents they could use in service to their family and friends as adults. Since Charles was an excellent student, they explained that they wanted to enrich his schooling by supporting development of his additional talents.

Then Charles presented his rationale about being a member of the set crew. He could refine his carpentry and visual arts skills, which his father had nurtured early on when they built a family room onto their home. He could experience the arts from behind the scenes; music, drama, and art were very important contributions to his mother. Charles wove in the information about his commitment with validating his parents for the gifts they gave him and wanted to develop further.

Charles's parents asked a lot of questions, and moved from anxiety to anticipation of Charles's desire to develop interests that they valued. Charles emphasized the hard work, peoples' reliance on him, and the service he could perform for his community— the school. These were all important family values, so Charles was able to show his parents he wasn't abandoning their family by doing this new activity. The play director invited the parents to stop by any time they were working to see the progress, and told about family get-togethers with the cast and crew during the production.

When the play came around, Charles's entire family—uncles, aunts, cousins alike— came to the performances. They sent playbills home to their native land showing Charles's name as the set crew carpenter. They also came to tell the occupational therapist and play director how grateful they were that people took a personal interest in their son's development.

This case illustrates an important and expanded role for occupational therapist's serving children in schools. We do not need to limit our expertise to children with identified disabilities. Other people also have participation challenges that can be addressed with the expertise of the occupational therapist. In this case, the occupational therapist's ability to respect cultural norms, family dynamics, and the contextual opportunities yielded a quality life experience for a young man finding his way. Isn't this always our calling?

Case Study #3 Learning Activity R

What if Charles was from a White family who supported his participation as long as he paid for the gas to get to and from practices and work days? What would change about your data-gathering strategies and the intervention options you might offer to Charles? Go through this same process with your classmates and design some plans for Charles with this change in the story. Discuss what issues might affect Charles's ability to be successful, what the characteristics of tasks are, what Charles's plans might look like, and how the contexts might help or create barriers for him. Then develop some conceptually based hypotheses and recommendations for Charles that are respectful of the family situation.

Summary

Using the EHP model and its associated terminology, occupational therapists can focus on all the possibilities for a person's life. We set our sights on participation for all individuals and communities. We also consider how satisfied people are with their participation in key contexts in their lives. Therapists give equal consideration to the person's skills and abilities, the context, and the tasks to decide how to facilitate better and more satisfying participation in life. Supports and barriers to participation are different for everyone and the EHP model offers intervention options to guide the process of deciding what to do to support participation.

When we focus on the person factors and the context, we become leaders in supporting inclusion. We offer our team members a vision of what is possible to support children who are different in some ways, and we help them see these children are like their peers in other ways. We stop thinking about disability and start thinking about children. The more we can understand how to adjust environments and tasks, the more it will be possible to include everyone all the time. With the generic language, EHP also invites interdisciplinary collaboration with the common goal of supporting all possible ways to get a successful outcome.

References

American Occupational Therapy Association. (2002). Occupational therapy practice framework: Domain and process. *American Journal of Occupational Therapy, 56,* 609-639.

Bulgren, J. A., Gilbert, M. P., Hall, J., Horton, B., Mellard, D., & Parker, K. (1997). *Accommodating adults with disabilities in adult education programs: National field test.* University of Kansas Institute for Adult Studies.

Christiansen, C., & Baum, C. (1997). Understanding occupation: Definitions and concepts. In C. Christiansen & C. Baum (Eds.), *Occupational therapy: Enabling function and well-being* (pp. 2-25). Thorofare, NJ: SLACK Incorporated.

Clark, R., Parham, D., Carlson, M., Frank, G., Jackson, J., Pierce, D., Wolfe, R. J., & Zemke, R. (1991). Occupational science: Academic innovation in the service of occupational therapy's future. *American Journal of Occupational Therapy, 45,* 300-310.

Dunn, W., Brown, C., & McGuigan, A. (1994). The ecology of human performance: A framework for considering the effect of context. *American Journal of Occupational Therapy, 48*(7), 595-607.

Dunn, W., Youngstrom, M., & Brown, C. (2003). Ecological model of occupation. In P. Kramer, J. Hinojosa, & C. B. Royeen (Eds.), *Perspectives in human occupation: Participation in life.* Baltimore: Lippincott, Williams & Wilkins.

Nelson, D. L. (1996). Therapeutic occupation: A definition. *American Journal of Occupational Therapy, 50,* 775-782.

Teel, C., Dunn, W., Jackson, S., & Duncan, P. (1997). The role of the environment in fostering independence: Conceptual and methodological issues in developing an instrument. *Topics in Stroke Rehabilitation, 4*(1), 28-40.

7

USING OCCUPATION BY DESIGN TO SYNTHESIZE ACROSS MULTIPLE MODELS FOR SERVICES TO CHILDREN AND FAMILIES

Christine Teeters Myers, MHS, OTR/L; Shirley O'Brien, MS, OTR/L, FAOTA; Doris Pierce, PhD, OTR/L, FAOTA; and Mary Ellen Thompson, MS, OTR/L

Learning Objectives

At the end of this chapter, the reader will be able to:
- Identify and understand key concepts of the Occupation by Design approach.
- Analyze multiple models from the Occupation by Design approach.
- Apply the Occupation by Design approach to a case example.
- Identify future practice and research opportunities.

Synthesizing Across Multiple Models for Family-Centered Occupational Therapy

Occupational therapy offers multiple approaches upon which a practitioner can draw in providing family-centered care. In this book, the following frames of reference and models have been featured:
- Sensory Integration (SI) and Neurodevelopmental Treatment (NDT)
- Person-Environment-Occupation (PEO) model
- Model of Human Occupation (MOHO)
- Occupational Adaptation (OA)
- Ecology of Human Performance (EHP)

How is a therapist to integrate the different perspectives provided by these approaches? How do they become a part of clinical reasoning in order to be implemented in family-centered services? How can we ensure that we provide interventions that are family centered and occupation based? In this chapter, we will synthesize across the multiple approaches provided in the book through several steps: 1) reviewing the clinical reasoning processes of occupational therapists, 2) considering each approach within the broad perspective of Occupation by Design (Pierce, 2001, 2003), 3) comparing the approaches, and 4) providing a case that demonstrates the implementation of different approaches by different therapists as a child transitions from one phase of services to another.

CLINICAL REASONING RESEARCH IN OCCUPATIONAL THERAPY

As we consider how the models offered in this book are useful for assisting children and families, it is important to understand how therapists think. Despite all our frames of reference and models, therapists' thinking about the therapy they provide is unique to each individual therapist. No two therapists reason alike.

Clinical reasoning research in occupational therapy is largely built on Donald Schon's theories of reflective practice (1983; Unsworth, 2005). Schon studied the use of tacit knowledge and technical rationality by experienced practitioners. He described *reflection-in-action* as the continual consideration of one's own thinking and problem solving while engaged in intervention. Although highly skilled, this process is difficult for experienced therapists to articulate. As Joan Rogers paraphrased Schon in her 1983 Slagle Lecture, "Expert clinicians are those who are competent in action and, simultaneously, reflect on this action to learn from it" (p. 616). In a study of clinical reasoning in psychosocial group practice, Ward (2003) described the therapist's awareness of his or her own thinking and behavior in relation to the client as "horizons on a field of consciousness...the phrase used by phenomenologists for...sensitivity to one's inner and outer world" (p. 630).

Based on Schon's theories, the first large scale study of clinical reasoning in occupational therapy was completed in the 1980s. Cheryl Mattingly, a student of Schon's, and Maureen Fleming, an accomplished occupational therapy researcher in her own right, teamed up to study occupational therapy reasoning, with support from the American Occupational Therapy Foundation. Together, they identified occupational therapy's use of procedural, interactive, conditional, and narrative forms of reasoning (Fleming, 1991; Mattingly, 1991; Mattingly & Fleming, 1994). Their findings, published in book form, remain the primary body of work on clinical reasoning in occupational therapy.

Later, Schell and Cervero (1993) expanded on Mattingly's and Fleming's conceptualization by suggesting that the types of occupational therapy reasoning included scientific reasoning (similar to procedural), narrative reasoning (interactive and conditional), and pragmatic reasoning. Schell and Cervero's new addition, pragmatic reasoning, was the thinking of therapists as they took into account the constraints and limitations beyond the therapist-client interaction and within which they provided intervention. Pragmatic reasoning recognizes factors such as reimbursement, access to equipment and space, necessary supports, therapist skills, and department traditions of intervention. Schell and Cervero echoed the concerns of Neuhaus (1988) in regard to the shaping of intervention by cost controls and new technology. They also emphasized the need to better understand the motivations and personal paradigms of therapists as they practice. Hooper (1997) later described the influence of the therapist's worldview on clinical reasoning, postulating that clinical rationales were rooted in the dynamic relationship between the therapist's treatment approach and his or her underlying life philosophy.

Most recently, Unsworth (2005) identified generalization reasoning, the use of therapists' experiences to frame and design treatment for clients similar to those to whom they have previously provided services. The reliance of therapists on their own experiences and that of other therapists in making judgments regarding intervention was earlier described by Rogers (1983) in her Eleanor Clark Slagle Lecture. Although clinicians rely on formal theories, they must often make decisions that depend on knowledge gained through experience (Javetz & Katz, 1989).

Generally, all types of clinical reasoning are implemented in overlapping and simultaneous ways, rather than as a single exclusive mode used at a particular time. Schon's work spurred parallel research in many fields, including physical therapy (Clouder, 2000), medicine (Lagerlov, Loeb, Andrew, & Hjortdahl, 2000), and nursing (Graham, 2000; Paget, 2001). Related aspects of current understandings of clinical reasoning in occupational therapy include research on ethical reasoning, the reasoning of novices vs. experts, and teaching clinical reasoning (Unsworth, 2005). In summary, many different terms have been used to describe the thinking of therapists: reflection, decision making, problem solving, design, and clinical reasoning (Mattingly & Fleming, 1994; Pierce, 2001, 2003; Schell & Cervero, 1993; Schon, 1983). Understanding therapists' clinical reasoning as a fluid and experiential process gives us a basis for understanding how therapists can best apply the models offered here to support family-centered care.

THE UNIQUE CLINICAL REASONING OF PEDIATRIC OCCUPATIONAL THERAPISTS THAT SUPPORTS OCCUPATION-BASED, FAMILY-CENTERED PRACTICE

Occupational therapists providing service delivery to pediatric populations have long understood the value of having client-centered, family-based approaches to the intervention needs of children and families. It is difficult to work effectively with children without being highly interactive with the child's family. Public laws affecting infants, children, and their families further reinforce the need to focus on occupation, environment, and needs for participation in occupation. Occupational therapists in pediatrics have offered services incorporating the child, his or her family, the context/environment, and occupation comfortably for the past 30 years (Reilly, 1974). The emphasis on play that is required to practice occupational therapy with children has also kept pediatric occupational therapy close to its roots in occupation. Thus, pediatric occupational therapists are well-positioned to lead the implementation of family-centered intervention.

Research on clinical reasoning focuses on the thinking processes of health care providers. These are not processes unique to occupational therapy. What differentiates between fields is not the type of clinical reasoning used, but the unique professional knowledge with which practitioners reason as they provide care. To describe to occupational therapists how to use unique professional concepts in practice, we have conceptual models such as those presented in this book. Most occupational therapy models do, more or less directly, focus on the profession's primary modality: occupation. But each model brings this out in a very different way. Therapists must choose when to use one model or another, and how to try to combine these approaches to make the most of their strengths.

How are we to contrast the differences in what each model offers? In this synthesizing chapter, we will use the broad lens of Occupation by Design to see how each of the approaches offered in the foregoing chapters shapes occupation-based intervention with children and families.

THE OCCUPATION BY DESIGN APPROACH

Occupation by Design is a broad model of how occupation is used in practice (Pierce, 2001, 2003). It rests on the therapist's sophisticated understanding and application of the

Figure 7-1. Occupation by Design circles. (From Pierce, D. E.: *Occupation by design: Building therapeutic power.* F.A. Davis Co., Philadelphia, 2003, pp. 3, 9, with permission.)

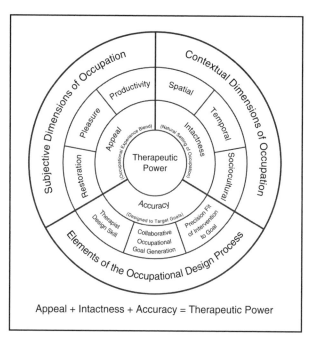

Appeal + Intactness + Accuracy = Therapeutic Power

typical and individually unique occupational nature of human beings. This approach targets therapeutically powerful interventions through the therapist's knowledge of occupations in context, combined with the therapist's skills for designing highly accurate interventions. In order to be effective in applying a particular occupation, the therapist must understand the occupation's general history, developmental variations, cultural meanings, contexts, and specific meaning to his or her client. This is why students in occupational therapy programs often study typical occupations separately from intervention.

In recent years, occupational science has emerged to address the need of occupational therapists to more deeply understand occupation. Surgeons study anatomy and physiology before they attempt surgery. Pharmacists study chemistry prior to learning to dispense medications. Similarly, occupational therapists need to understand occupation prior to using it as intervention. Of course, for many years, occupational therapy has not had a well-developed basic science of its own. Sometimes, having done well so far without this foundation, we wonder why we need it. This is a natural dynamic in the maturation of the discipline and the profession. In future years, the field will wonder how we could have practiced without a basic science, just as medicine now looks back in wonder on its practice prior to the work of the early anatomists. The better the therapist's understanding of occupation, the more effective he or she will be in selecting occupations that are appealing to a particular client or family and in working with them to accurately identify valued occupational goals.

The Occupation by Design process rests on four primary questions (Figure 7-1):

1. What is the occupational nature of this client?

2. What therapeutic occupations may appeal to this person?

3. In what context are they appealing?

4. What occupations are problematic and may be addressed as goals?

The dynamics of the Occupation by Design approach is most easily overviewed through this circular model that targets, at its center, the therapeutic power of the intervention. Therapeutic power emanates from several sources:

- The appeal to the client of the blend of productivity, pleasure, and/or restoration during the therapeutic occupation
- The contextual intactness (or naturalness) to the client of the place, time, and people involved in the therapeutic occupation
- The therapist's skills of design, collaborative goal setting, and creation of a close fit between intervention and goal

Appeal

The higher the appeal to the client of a therapeutic occupation, the more effective it will be. We have all, as therapists, experienced the wide range of responses that clients can have to intervention, from excitement and fun during therapy to downright boredom and resistance. To provide highly appealing interventions, we must make judgments about the occupational nature of our client and then select therapeutic occupations that are appealing to that person. If we consider the family as our client, then we must similarly consider the occupational nature of that family as an entity and select therapeutic occupations that are appealing to them. Sometimes a balance must be struck between what is appealing to the child and what is appealing to the family.

Appeal comes from the combined pleasurable, productive, and restorative aspects of an occupation. For children, high appeal often depends on creating therapeutic occupations that are highly pleasurable because they are sensory, playful, active, or fun. These characteristics can be very appealing to the whole family and have always been central to occupational therapy for children. Using productivity to increase appeal for the family and child might be done through feelings of challenge, arousal, flow, accomplishment, craftsmanship, pride in a product or outcome, or positive worker or student identities. To use restoration to strengthen appeal, the therapist would attend to sleeping and eating in the family's life and might include in therapeutic occupations the characteristics of restfulness, calm energy levels, enjoyment of food and drink, self-care and quiet focus activities, nature, and spirituality.

Thus, to enhance the appeal of a therapeutic occupation for a child and his or her family, you might consider the following questions:

- What blend of productivity, pleasure, and restoration will provide the most appealing and effective therapeutic occupations for this child and family?
- What highly productive occupations might serve as interventions?
- What highly pleasurable occupations might serve as interventions?
- What highly restorative occupations might serve as interventions?
- Are different family members different in terms of these needs?

Intactness

The more intact, or natural, the context of the therapeutic occupation is, the more powerful it will be. That is, the therapeutic occupation will be effective only to the degree that it occurs in the usual time, place, and social setting it would if it was not being used as therapy. Intactness is not always fully possible, due to constraints on service delivery. However, therapists can always find ways to more closely approximate full intactness by making changes to the spatial, temporal, and social contexts in which they offer therapy. This makes therapy feel more natural to the family and supports their full involvement, as well as increases generalization.

There are four primary modes for making the context of intervention more intact. The most obvious way to make therapy more intact for families and children is to deliver it within "their" contexts—their homes, schools, and neighborhoods—instead of a clinic or center. Being in the natural settings of children and families offers unexpected therapy resources, makes families and children more comfortable, increases generalization, and helps to make the child and family more fully participatory partners on the care team. Another way to enhance intactness is to make supportive modifications to the environments in which children and their families live and work. Sometimes you may select a therapy setting that is novel for the child and family because of the unique activities offered there, such as karate class, Cub Scouts, a stable, or a community pool. Lastly, the settings in which therapists work can be naturalized by making them more like culturally appropriate home and school settings instead of bright-white medical clinics full of strange and scary-looking equipment.

Intactness has three dimensions: spatial, temporal, and sociocultural.

- To enhance the intactness of the spatial context of interventions, consider especially the client-environment interface through vision and the hand, environmental qualities of sound and safety and crowding, way-finding, ergonomics, tools and toys, and public vs. private space.

- To enhance the intactness of the temporal context, consider the circadian rhythms of children and their families, usual calendars, cultural differences in time use, orchestration of activities, memory, routines, narratives, and developmental sequences.

- To enhance the intactness of the sociocultural context, consider the difference in perspectives of therapists and clients, personal identities of the child and family, solitary vs. shared occupations, key relationships, organizations in which clients and their families are involved, meaningful rituals, diversity, and gender.

Most importantly, ensure that clients and their families remain the primary decision makers in therapy.

Thus, to enhance the intactness of a therapeutic occupation for a child and his or her family, you might consider the following questions:

- What settings do this child and family usually occupy during a usual week and weekend?

- In what aspects of these usual settings are there problems?

- Are there settings in which treatment might be offered, thus making interventions more intact for this child and family?

- What spatial characteristics of intervention might be changed to enhance intactness?

- What temporal characteristics of intervention might be changed to enhance intactness?

- What sociocultural characteristics of interventions might be changed to enhance intactness?

Accuracy

To enhance the therapeutic power of occupation-based practice through increased accuracy, the therapist requires strong skills of creative design, collaborative occupational goal generation, and intervention/goal fit.

Occupational therapists vary in the degree to which their creative abilities are developed. Some come from art backgrounds that give them skills with color, form, and texture. These are not, however, the creative skills emphasized in the Occupation by Design approach. For occupational therapists, the professional-level design skills required to maximize treatment effects include seven skills: 1) personal motivation, 2) information seeking and analysis, 3) defining projects and needs clearly, 4) dependably and quickly generating a large number of solutions for any challenge, 5) careful selection of best plans to meet specific criteria, 6) complex and flexible implementations, and 7) reflective evaluation of all interventions and programming.

Collaborative occupational goal generation is central to working with children and families. We must ensure that those with whom we work feel ownership of therapy directions and are welcome to guide interventions in the directions they see as most needed. We must be great interviewers, skilled at hearing and valuing the story our clients and their families tell of their journeys and their hoped-for destinations.

Selecting therapeutic occupations that best respond to collaborative goals with a close fit requires attentiveness, observation, resourcefulness, perseverance, and experience. No session is perfect, but some are more effective than others.

Thus, to enhance the accuracy of a therapeutic occupation for a child and his or her family, you might consider the following questions.

- Within the seven phases of design skills listed above, what are your own strengths and weaknesses? What skills might you improve to enhance the accuracy of your interventions?

- Are your assessments truly collaborative and open to shared goal setting with families? Do the children and families with whom you work own and guide the interventions you provide? Are you short circuiting your therapeutic power by depending more heavily on therapist judgment to select goals and less on family input?

- Are your interview and observation skills at research competency levels?

- Are you resourceful in creating occupation-based interventions that provide a close match with the goals valued by the child and family?

- What occupations are most problematic for this family and child?

- What occupational goals would they like to select?

According to the elements of a model posited by Dunbar in Chapter 1, Occupation by Design is structured by the aspects described in Table 7-1.

In the following section, Occupation by Design is used to structure exploration of the different models for working with families and children that are presented in the chapters of this book. By using the core concepts of appeal, intactness, and accuracy from Occupation by Design, it is possible to compare the models in terms of the different tools they offer to therapists. As has been demonstrated in clinical reasoning research, experienced therapists do not reason solely from a single model, but from an integrative perspective that comes from multiple models and theories, interactions with the client and family, and past experiences of providing services to similar clients.

Viewing Different Approaches Through Occupation by Design

THE SENSORY INTEGRATION AND NEURODEVELOPMENTAL TREATMENT FRAMES OF REFERENCES

The SI frame of reference posits that human beings are driven to seek out sensory stimulation to receive optimal sensory nourishment. Adequate sensory processing allows children to participate in the everyday occupations of childhood. An occupational therapist utilizing a SI approach might ask, "What lack or immaturity of sensory integration is interfering with a child's ability to participate?" The NDT frame of reference looks more

Table 7-1

THE ELEMENTS OF OCCUPATION BY DESIGN AS A PRACTICE MODEL

Philosophical Assumptions	Humans are occupational beings. They express and develop their identities and place in the world through doing.
Ethics	Occupational therapy is best provided in a client-centered, collaborative style that respects and custom designs to match the individuality of each client.
Theoretical Foundation	A wide variety of theories are used to describe occupation, drawing from the discipline of occupational science as well as other disciplines.
Domain of Concern	Explication of occupation in order to better understand clients as occupational beings, set occupational goals, and apply occupation as the primary modality of the profession is the domain of concern.
Nature/Principles for Sequencing Aspects of Practice	Appeal, intactness, and accuracy of therapeutic occupations are used to meet collaboratively set occupational goals.
Legitimate Tools	Tools include knowledge of typical and individual occupation, therapeutic occupational experiences, collaborative occupational goal setting, and therapeutic design process.

specifically at the development of normal muscle tone, reflexive responses, and movement patterns to allow a child to participate in his or her preferred occupations. Using NDT, one might ask, "What abnormal muscle tone or motor skills are interfering with a child's ability to participate?" The pediatric occupational therapist with training in these frames of reference will assess how these basic neurological functions are interfering with the child's productive, pleasurable, and restorative occupations.

Appeal in the Sensory Integration and Neurodevelopmental Treatment Frames of Reference

The child's ability to integrate sensory information from his or her body and environment can directly affect the ability to engage in occupations that are productive, pleasurable, and restorative. Infants' and toddlers' primary productive activity is exploring their environment. Preschoolers often work hard at play and start to help with household activities, such as picking up their toys. School-aged children need to attend school and complete homework and may have very goal-centered after school activities. For young children, pleasure is intertwined with productivity. Without normal integration of sensory input, pleasure may not be possible. A soft caress is not a pleasant experience for a child who is tactilely defensive.

Sleeping, eating and drinking, self-care activities, and quiet focus activities are occupations that allow us to restore our physical and mental selves. Restoration is critical to productive and pleasurable occupations. Since SI affects arousal level, poor regulation may lead to a multitude of sleep issues—poor quality of sleep, inadequate sleep, the need to sleep at inappropriate times, or the hyperactivity and irritability that typically results from tiredness in children.

Tactile defensiveness may severely limit the variety of foods a child will eat. Poor tactile and proprioceptive processing can contribute to an inadequate ability to eat or drink by mouth. Decreased vestibular function may affect attention to task and/or the muscle tone needed for self-feeding and other daily activities. Neurodevelopmental problems may require an excess of energy output in order to accomplish everyday tasks. This will increase the need for daily restoration.

Questions on using the SI frame of reference to create appealing therapeutic occupations:

- Is oversensitivity to tactile input preventing an infant from crawling very far or from placing interesting objects into his or her mouth for exploration?
- Is a lack of proprioceptive processing interfering with a school-aged child's development of handwriting that is legible and quick?
- Is poor vestibular processing interfering with accurate visual perception?
- What therapeutic occupations may appeal to this child and family, in view of his or her sensory processing issues?

Questions on using the NDT frame of reference to create appealing therapeutic occupations:

- Is lack of muscle tone preventing an infant from developing the shoulder and hip stability necessary for crawling?
- Is retention of immature reflexes interfering with the child's ability to maintain the eye gaze needed for tracking an object or to have a stable seated position for handwriting?
- What therapeutic occupations may appeal to this child and family, in view of any irregular muscle tone or motor limitations?

Intactness in the Sensory Integration and Neurodevelopmental Treatment Frames of Reference

SI affects the child's ability to interact with the environment. Children learn about the spatial aspects of their environment through vision, physical interaction, mobile exploration, and fine motor skills. Poor integration of visual input will interfere with the child's ability to build an accurate spatial understanding of the environment. Temporally, poor sensory processing can lead to irregular biorhythms. Habits and routines may be particularly difficult to establish. A child who does not eat or sleep on a regular schedule also disrupts the family's routine. Similarly, a child who takes an inordinate amount of time to complete daily activities such as dressing and eating will also disrupt the family's day.

The child with SI dysfunction can have socially unacceptable behaviors, such as an inability to sit still, an overly loud voice, or a tendency to bite. He or she may not be able to participate in cultural activities such as attending church. The child may have difficulty forming friendships. The child may be ostracized from shared occupations, like going to the movies or watching television. It can be particularly distressing to other family members if the child is unable to participate in what the family considers to be important occupations that express who they are and the culture to which they belong.

Questions on using the SI frame of reference to create intact therapeutic occupations:

- Can the treatment activity occur in the usual space for this occupation?

- How can the spatial, temporal, or social aspects of the environment be modified to help facilitate better sensory processing, as well as feelings of competency and success?

- Does this child bite others?

- Is he or she able to participate in a group activity without covering his or her ears and screaming?

- Is he or she likely to tell someone that person smells badly and start gagging?

Questions on using the NDT frame of reference to create intact therapeutic occupations:

- How is lack of mobility due to abnormal neuromotor development interfering with the child's ability to explore the environment?

- Are abnormal muscle tone, poor shoulder stability, lack of trunk and neck control, or retention of abnormal reflexes interfering with the child's ability to effectively direct his or her hands toward interaction with the environment?

- How can the spatial, temporal, or social aspects of the environment be modified to help facilitate better muscle tone and movement, as well as feelings of competency and success?

Accuracy in the Sensory Integration and Neurodevelopmental Treatment Frames of Reference

The occupational therapist should start with a thorough understanding of the family's typical day, the timing and rhythm of daily occupations. Any therapeutic activities should fit into this rhythm and aim toward normalizing the family day. Dressing, for example, is a typical daily occupation that a child with SI dysfunction may have difficulty completing. First, assess what parts of dressing are difficult for the child. Then, develop as many ideas as possible about activities that address these issues. Finally, narrow some of these ideas to fit what you know about this family's routine.

Whether you are using SI, an NDT approach, or both together, consider how your work fits within the family's goals. Some parents want to have their child rapidly progress to self-dressing without a lot of concern for style or neatness. Other parents may wish to retain more control of the dressing but want the processes to be less time consuming and less of a battle with the child. Some parents may wish to understand how they might help their child dress in a way that does not encourage abnormal reflexes and muscle tone. After each treatment session, consider how the next treatment will reflect the change (Table 7-2).

Questions on using the SI frame of reference to create accurate therapeutic occupations:

- What occupations do the family and child feel are being most disrupted by the child's sensory processing issues?

- How well have you fit the SI approach into the family routine? Are there tactile issues with the feel of the clothing, proprioceptive issues with the amount of pressure needed to pull up a zipper?

- Can the child tolerate a more challenging piece of clothing—jeans vs. sweat pants?

- Is the family routine changing as the child's ability to process sensory information improves?

Questions on using the NDT frame of reference to create accurate therapeutic occupations:

Table 7-2

APPEAL, INTACTNESS, AND ACCURACY FOR
SENSORY INTEGRATION AND NEURODEVELOPMENTAL TREATMENT

Occupation by Design	Sensory Integration/NDT
Appeal	The child's sensory integrative and neurodevelopmental abilities have a direct impact on the appeal of an occupation.
Intactness	The goodness of fit in the interaction between the child and the environment in which the occupation is occurring.
Accuracy	Collaborative goal setting with the family considers the child's sensory and neurodevelopmental needs.

- What occupations do the family and child feel are being most disrupted by the child's neurodevelopmental challenges?
- How well have you fit the NDT treatment into the family routine?
- Are the parents comfortable with the NDT handling techniques taught to them?
- Is the child's muscle tone so high that it makes it difficult to put on his or her pants?
- Can he or she maintain pinch long enough to pull up his or her own zipper?

THE PERSON-ENVIRONMENT-OCCUPATION MODEL

The PEO model focuses on the transactional nature of the interaction between the person, his or her environment, and his or her occupations. The PEO model is fairly congruent with Occupation by Design. Person, environment, and occupations interact across time and space in such a way as to either increase or decrease the goodness of fit between the three. The PEO model describes tasks, activities, and occupations as nested one within the other. A multitude of tasks make up an activity and a multitude of activities make up an occupation. This is somewhat different than Occupation by Design. In Occupation by Design, an activity is a cultural idea about doing, allowing for general communication about occupations. Occupations are specific experiences that are personally constructed, spatially located, and not repeatable. The PEO model takes a more traditional approach to balance, dividing activities into the categories of self-care, productivity, and leisure. Occupation by Design more broadly defines balance as a pattern of occupations that blends pleasure, productivity, and restoration within occupations and in a way that is satisfying to a particular individual.

Appeal in the Person-Environment-Occupation Model

The PEO model views the person as a complex combination of specific characteristics and life experiences. For an occupation to appeal, it must address these complexities with a balance of pleasure, productivity, and restoration. Appeal for children will change as they mature and develop. Very young children primarily are interested in pleasure and restoration. As they reach school age, productivity takes a stronger place in appeal of occupations. The specific characteristics of the child need to be considered in deciding which occupations will appeal.

Table 7-3

APPEAL, INTACTNESS, AND ACCURACY FOR
THE PERSON-ENVIRONMENT-OCCUPATION MODEL

Occupation by Design	Person-Environment-Occupation Model
Appeal	The unique characteristics of the child contribute to the appeal of an occupation for that child.
Intactness	The environment (i.e., contexts and situations outside the child) is key to intactness.
Accuracy	Occupational performance is a result of the match between the child, the environment, and the occupation.

Questions on using the PEO model to create appealing therapeutic occupations:
- What are the child's personal characteristics (such as cognitive function, physical abilities, or emotional abilities) that affect his or her ability to participate in an occupation?
- What life experiences have influenced the child's preferred occupations?
- What activities would appeal to this child and family?

Intactness in the Person-Environment-Occupation Model

Environment includes cultural, social, physical, and institutional aspects that may contain barriers or supports to performance of occupations. Occupations allow a person to meet his or her need for self-maintenance, expression, and fulfillment as defined by the PEO model. Environment is key to the intactness of an occupation. For this reason, children under the age of 3 are treated in their home environment. Once a child is preschool-aged, the treatment focus changes to the school environment. It is important to not lose sight of all the environments in which a child engages in occupational performances. For example, a grade school child may spend time at the local park or in after school activities. It is important that occupational therapists advocate for a child's access to all pertinent age-appropriate and valued environments.

Questions on using the PEO model to create intact therapeutic occupations:
- Are there occupations specific to this child's culture in which they are unable to participate?
- What aspects of the environment can be changed to encourage participation in typical childhood occupations?
- In what settings would it be most effective to offer treatment to this child and family?

Accuracy in the Person-Environment-Occupation Model

Occupational performances are both objective (observable) and subjective. They are affected by the transaction between the person, environment, and occupation. Maximizing the fit between these three aspects of occupational performance strengthens the accuracy of the intervention. For accuracy, the occupational therapist needs to have a thorough understanding of the client's personal characteristics, of typical environments in which he or she performs occupations, and of the types of occupations in which the child would normally participate (Table 7-3).

Questions on using the PEO model to create accurate therapeutic occupations:
- What aspect of occupational performance can I best influence—the person, the environment, or the occupation?
- What areas of occupational performance would the family and child identify as most critical for goal setting?

THE MODEL OF HUMAN OCCUPATION

The MOHO uses general systems to explain the dynamics of occupation as it outputs to and receives feedback from the environment. This is one of the oldest of the models presented in this text. MOHO, first published in the 1980s, focused our thinking on occupation as intervention. This model does not emphasize the specific effectiveness of treatment, but rather is a broader conceptual model addressing the person and his or her efficacy and effectiveness within roles and habits in context.

MOHO has contributed greatly to understanding occupation in context through a commitment to instrument development. Many standardized assessments for use in practice have been initiated through the collaborative efforts of practitioners and academicians. Blending the dynamic nature of individual client interests, habits, and skills in context, practitioners can guide intervention planning using this model. The systematic approach to evaluation of children and families, based on key concepts in the model, has strengthened the model for intervention.

Appeal in the Model of Human Occupation

The dynamic components of volition clearly address the key aspects of appeal. Personal causation, values, and interests all contribute to identification of the pleasurable, productive, and restorative occupations of the child and the family. The volitional processes of anticipating, choosing, experiencing, and interpreting participation reinforce the child's understanding of competence and achievement as he or she engages in occupations. Thus, the child will choose to engage in a variety of occupations through which he or she gains pleasure, productivity, and restoration.

Habituation also incorporates the habits and roles that the infant, child, and his or her family experience. Family routines and rituals may enrich the appeal of occupations within temporal and physical contexts. Habits and roles may be viewed in terms of the appeal of the occupation, as well as the intactness.

The interrelationship of volition, habituation, and performance capacity is a dynamic and individualized experience for children and their families. The subjective experience of the lived body clearly links the child's performance capacity to the occupation pursued. It is through components of performance capacity that we are able to discern physical and mental aspects of participation in occupation.

Questions on using MOHO to create appealing therapeutic occupations:
- What occupations are of interest to the child and the family?
- How do these occupations fit into daily family routines?
- What habits and skills support the child's ability to participate in these occupations?

Intactness in the Model of Human Occupation

Volition and habituation are shaped by intactness. The temporal and sociocultural aspects of interests, personal causation, values, roles, and habits are intertwined with appeal. The child's engagement in the rhythm, intensity, and duration of contextual experiences also contributes to the appeal of the occupation. The childhood routines and opportunities are temporally shaped by the dynamic demands of the family.

Table 7-4
APPEAL, INTACTNESS, AND ACCURACY FOR
THE MODEL OF HUMAN OCCUPATION

Occupation by Design	Model of Human Occupation
Appeal	Appeal is demonstrated by the dynamic interaction of the child's volition, habituation, and performance capacity for participation in occupation. Appeal is subjective and shaped by individual child and family values and preferences.
Intactness	Intactness is observed through the shaping of occupation by the physical and social elements within which it occurs. Engagement in occupation reflects rhythm, intensity, and duration in a particular environment. Opportunity is reflected in physical and social environments.
Accuracy	Occupational participation, occupational performance, and skills all are viewed as important to accuracy. Participation and performance of occupations in natural environments best demonstrate the child's abilities.

The environment, as presented within MOHO, organizes our understanding of the physical and social elements that may shape the child's occupational experience. The social elements greatly affect the development of habits and routines in childhood. Family cultural practices may impact occupations that children actively participate in during a particular time period. The ways in which children participate in their environments relies on their ability to incorporate both appeal and intactness of occupations.

Questions on using MOHO to create intact therapeutic occupations:
- Where does the child participate in his or her chosen occupations?
- Who does the child participate with? When does this occur?
- What type of interaction and/or engagement is expected in the environment?
- What are the rhythm, intensity, and duration of preferred routines?
- What environmental modifications are necessary for successful participation in chosen routines?
- In what environments would intervention best be offered?
- How may sociocultural factors impact performance of routines and habits?

Accuracy in the Model of Human Occupation

Accuracy is a strength of MOHO. Through the commitment to instrument development, occupational therapists have access to reliable and valid tools to realize improved accuracy. The assessment tools recognize the dynamic interplay of an individual's values, interests, skills, routines, and habits in specific environments. Thus, the power of occupation is captured through measurement.

Accuracy, as conceptualized within Occupation by Design, is best observed in how the occupational therapist organizes and targets goals for intervention, in collaboration with the family and/or child in a given setting. Occupational participation blends the child's skill development with the demands experienced in natural occupations. The therapist must use design skills and collaborative planning to ensure precision in meeting intervention goals for both families and children (Table 7-4).

Questions on using MOHO to create accurate therapeutic occupations:

- What assessments would best elicit understanding of the child's desires for participation in occupation? Opportunities for engagement?
- What assessments best capture the child's/family's values and preferences about childhood habits and routines and occupational performance?
- How can we collaborate with families to best address the intervention needs of the child?

THE OCCUPATIONAL ADAPTATION MODEL

OA offers a strong emphasis on client centeredness along with the skills of the child and his or her family. The OA model offers further insights into how a child engages in productive, pleasurable, and restorative occupations. The concepts of effectiveness and press for mastery offer guidance for discussing and blending the role expectations of children with disabilities in particular contexts. In this model, the person is the one to make the necessary changes/adaptations. This may help in setting goals with families and other professionals involved in the usual contexts of their daily activities.

Appeal in the Occupational Adaptation Model

The blend of occupational experiences based on productive, pleasurable, and restorative occupations is strong in the OA model. The productivity of the child is considered as we look at the interaction between occupational challenges and his or her personal skills (cognitive, psychosocial, and sensorimotor). The match of expectations and skills in the area of adaptive response mechanisms will demonstrate how effectively and efficiently the child is able to participate in productive occupations. Reaching the goal presented by the occupational challenge provides feelings of productivity and accomplishment. The energy the child uses in a role (e.g., student) further demonstrates his or her abilities to engage in expected environments.

The concept of pleasure is one that comes naturally when discussing children. Pleasure is attained in this model when the child's desire for mastery and the press for mastery are supported by adaptive skills needed to attain the occupational challenge. Again, the environmental context contributes as the child experiences various sensations in the context.

Restoration is an important aspect in child and family development. Within the OA model, restoration is needed to allow the evaluative processes the time and the environment necessary for integration of learning. This learning occurs within the person. If adaptation processes are disorganized, the integrative process will be hampered. For example, if a child is constantly using primary energy requiring a high degree of focus, and always moving between too many projects (hypermobile) not making effective decisions, then his or her ability to integrate occupational challenges presented within the environment may be hampered.

Questions on using the OA model to create appealing therapeutic occupations:

- Does the child enjoy the therapeutic occupation?
- How can pleasure be maximized within a press for mastery?
- What type of energy is the child using primarily?
- Is the energy level supporting engagement in the particular context for the role expectations of the occupational challenge?
- Are families using adaptive response modes that foster productive occupations, through the use of routines and rituals?
- What does the child do to recharge body and mind?
- When is the child's down time? The family's down time?

- What routines and rituals are used within the family to help reinforce restoration?
- What sleep cycles are usual in the family? How are these reinforced through environment and routines?

Intactness in the Occupational Adaptation Model

Contextual dimensions are rich in the OA model. The therapist must give consideration to the various types of environments and strive to incorporate natural environments for treatment. By fostering engagement in occupations in natural environments, children are able to experience the occupational challenges inherent in the established environments. As families are involved in therapeutic interventions, incorporating natural environments allows for the facilitation of therapeutic power through occupations typical for both families and children.

Although the environment in this model is seen as relatively stable, it is the development of coping strategies and/or personal adaptation that affords both families and children the ability to integrate learning, as they attain occupational role expectations and respond to the press for mastery.

Questions on using the OA model to create intact therapeutic occupations:
- What are the natural environments in which this child engages in occupations?
- How do the environments support and/or constrain participation in occupations?
- What occupational challenges are presented to the child and family by the environment?
- How is the press for mastery of occupations impacted by the environment?

Accuracy in the Occupational Adaptation Model

Accuracy is the aspect of OA that fits most clearly with Occupation by Design. In the OA model, the therapist works in concert with the family and the child to effectively use existing and emerging skills to accomplish therapeutic interventions in natural contexts. Through engagement in structured problem-solving and decision-making processes based on occupational challenges, the child and family have the opportunity to experience guided learning in a safe environment. The occupational therapist uses the intactness of the environment for therapeutic fit, thus enhancing the therapeutic power of the intervention. Goals are collaboratively set, with refinement and precision coming from the client's desire for mastery and the therapist's knowledge about occupational responses and challenges. Accuracy is further reinforced through evaluative processes inherent in the individual's problem-solving and decision-making abilities. The therapist using OA structures engagements in occupations that will provide opportunities for self-evaluation by families and children (Table 7-5).

Questions on using the OA model to create accurate therapeutic occupations:
- What occupational challenges would the child and family like to choose as goals?
- What strategies does the child use to support occupational performance?
- How does the child respond to internal and external feedback about his or her participation in occupation?
- What coping skills are used by the child and/or family? Are they effective?

Table 7-5

APPEAL, INTACTNESS, AND ACCURACY FOR
THE OCCUPATIONAL ADAPTATION MODEL

Occupation by Design	*Occupational Adaptation Model*
Appeal	Appeal is heavily emphasized in the following concepts: person, adaptive response, adaptation energy, adaptation response modes, and behaviors. The uniqueness of the occupation to a child and family is shaped through the understanding of these concepts.
Intactness	The environment is extremely powerful in this model as the desire for mastery blends the challenges of the occupation in the natural environment with the child.
Accuracy	Adaptation captures the creative problem solving exhibited by the child, the family, and the therapist. Evaluation of specific outcomes and responses to engagement in occupation helps to refine occupational performance in the natural context.

THE ECOLOGY OF HUMAN PERFORMANCE MODEL

A shared focus on context results in many similarities between Occupation by Design and the EHP model. Both take into account the complexity and nonlinearity of human interactions within context, which is similarly conceptualized as including spatial/physical, temporal, and sociocultural characteristics. Interventions are perceived as having maximum potential and therapeutic value when carried out within the child's natural context. Both models support a client-centered approach in which intervention is developed through collaboration between the child, family, and therapist. Five proposed intervention strategies within the EHP model complement the clinical reasoning approach emphasized by Occupation by Design.

Appeal in the Ecology of Human Performance Model

The establish/restore intervention is a collaborative effort by the child, therapist, and family to remediate skills or learn new skills needed to support engagement in tasks. By focusing on the dimensions of productivity, pleasure, and restoration inherent in occupation, the skills become part of the occupational experience and thus more appealing for the child and family.

Questions on using the establish/restore strategy of the EHP to create appealing therapeutic occupations:

- What pleasurable, productive, and restorative occupations could also support specific skill development or remediation?

- How can families be involved in promoting skill development or remediation within occupations that are highly appealing for their child?

- In the adapt/modify intervention, the contextual features or the task characteristics are adjusted to support performance. A preschool-aged child who wants to participate in a coloring activity is inhibited by increased muscle tone. Through positioning in a chair that supports optimal posture and use of adapted writing implements, the child is able to color with the rest of his or her class. The adaptations allow him or her to remain engaged in an appealing occupational experience within the natural context of the classroom.

Questions on using the adapt/modify strategy of the EHP to create appealing therapeutic occupations:

- How can the context or task characteristics be adapted/modified to support the child's participation in the occupational experience?

- How can I best collaborate with the family to adapt/modify the context or task in order to sustain the same level of appeal or increase appeal of the desired occupation?

Intactness in the Ecology of Human Performance Model

In the establish/restore intervention, the child may appear to be the primary focus; however, the context remains an important aspect in this intervention. The more natural the context, the more likely skill development or relearning will occur. A mother's main concern for her 3-year-old daughter is her ability to participate in a weekly play group with other children. Rather than work on play skills in the home with only the therapist and the mother present, therapy occurs during the playgroup with the other children and their family members involved. By incorporating the occupation within its typical context, the occupational therapist makes the experience more intact.

Questions on using the establish/restore strategy of the EHP to create intact therapeutic occupations:

- How can the natural context of an occupation be used to support specific skill development or remediation?

- How can families participate in promoting their child's skill development or remediation within natural contexts?

- Which dimensions of context need to be altered: spatial/physical, temporal, or sociocultural?

Intactness is also relevant for the adapt/modify intervention. Even small adaptations in the environment may support performance and keep the occupational experience intact. A premature infant who has just come home from the hospital after a 2-month stay in the NICU may benefit from his or her family members making both spatial/physical and sociocultural adaptations to their home: modifying it to become a quiet and dimly lit space, rather than the typical state of the household—loud and bright.

Questions on using the adapt/modify strategy of the EHP to create intact therapeutic occupations:

- How can I best collaborate with the family to determine optimal contextual adaptations or modifications that will support the child's occupational engagement?

- Which dimensions of context need to be adapted/modified: spatial/physical, temporal, or sociocultural?

- Will potential adaptations/modifications decrease the level of intactness, sustain the same level of intactness, or increase the intactness of the desired occupation?

The alter intervention actually changes the context in which a task is to be enacted. The contextual dimensions of occupation that support intactness would be considered here. If the child is able to participate in a task, but the aspects of the context (spatial, temporal, or sociocultural) are not optimal for performance, the context may be changed, with the intent of simultaneously reinforcing participation and improving intactness. For instance, a 5-year-old child's favorite occupation is going for a walk with her father and the family dog, however, it is not safe to walk at night in the family's neighborhood. Perhaps the walk would be better taken in the morning, thus changing the temporal dimension of the context, or maybe there is a park nearby where they can walk the dog in the evenings, thus changing the spatial dimensions of the context. Either way, the child is able to engage in a meaningful occupational experience with her father and cherished pet.

Questions on using the alter strategy of the EHP to create intact therapeutic occupations:

- How can the context be altered while still leaving the occupation intact for the family and child?

- How can I best collaborate with the family to determine possible contextual alternatives for this occupation?

- What suggestions might the family have for alterations to the context of occupations?

Accuracy in the Ecology of Human Performance Model

When attempting to avert the occurrence of potential difficulties in performance, therapists may employ the preventive intervention. This intervention is supported in the Occupation by Design model through collaborative occupational goal generation. The therapist has specialized knowledge and experience that can benefit the child and family. This includes the ability to anticipate possible future occurrences that may be detrimental to the child's health and well-being and could be prevented. During collaborative occupational goal generation this concern could be made known to the family and addressed within the development of meaningful therapy goals.

Questions on using the prevent strategy of the EHP to create accurate therapeutic occupations:

- What information is necessary for the family to help support their understanding of possible future occurrences and how these relate to occupation?

- What is the best way to collaborate with families while developing goals aimed at preventing negative outcomes?

- How can specific prevent strategies be incorporated into daily routines in order to support family needs?

Establishing conditions that provide the foundations for the best possible performance is the purpose of the create intervention. This intervention is applicable to both individuals and populations, and does not require the assumption that a disability exists. Occupation by Design encompasses the create intervention through its emphasis on therapist design skill and approach to planning occupational experiences through client-therapist collaboration. An occupational therapist who works in an inclusive kindergarten classroom may create opportunities for all children in the classroom, not just those with disabilities, to engage in tasks that support handwriting development. Having the children choose a theme, write a word to describe parts of the theme, and illustrate their work incorporates collaboration between the therapist and the children while supporting inclusion of all children in an occupational experience (Table 7-6).

Questions on using the create strategy of the EHP to design accurate therapeutic occupations:

- What are the needs of the individual (child and/or family) or population?

- How can I collaborate with the individual (child and/or family) or population to determine the best ways to meet their needs?

- What is the optimal approach to collaborative goal setting within a population?

Table 7-6

APPEAL, INTACTNESS, AND ACCURACY FOR
THE ECOLOGY OF HUMAN PERFORMANCE MODEL

Occupation by Design	Ecology of Human Performance Model
Appeal	The process of establishing or restoring skills occurs as a part of the occupational experience, while adaptations or modifications support participation in appealing occupations within natural contexts.
Intactness	Occupations in natural contexts support skill development or remediation, while adaptation of the environment/task or alteration of contextual dimensions (spatial/physical, temporal, and/or sociocultural) may support participation in occupation.
Accuracy	Anticipation of possible future occurrences is linked to collaborative goal setting in order to prevent negative outcomes, while collaborative goal setting and therapist design skills create opportunities for engagement in occupations based on individual or population needs.

An Integrative Overview Across Approaches

Table 7-7 provides an overview of the five approaches offered in this book, integrated through the concepts of appeal, intactness, and accuracy, all drawn from Occupation by Design. Viewed in this way, different approaches have different strengths. The most long-lived models show the greatest dependence on extradisciplinary knowledge, yet have the most developed assessment instruments to support their use. Newer approaches tend to emphasize more strongly the environmental aspects of occupation and strategies for working with contextual dimension to enhance intervention impact. The more recently developed approaches also focus more on the conscious, subjective experience and meaning of occupations in intervention and in areas of disorganization and goal needs. There are many differences, as well as similarities, in the approaches.

Occupational therapy has matured rapidly in the past few decades. Instead of being faced with a lack of models that integrate extradisciplinary knowledge to support holistic, occupation-based practice, we are now faced with a wealth of choices and an emerging disciplinary knowledge base that more closely fits our practice needs. Luckily, there is no need to choose between the varieties of approaches to intervention. The reality of occupational therapists' clinical reasoning is that it is fluid, in the moment, multimodal, and draws on a blend of models to support judgment and interaction. All of the approaches presented here offer strengths to intervention. Together, they offer powerful therapeutic occupational outcomes for children and their families.

Table 7-7

An Integrative Overview Across Approaches Using Appeal, Intactness, and Accuracy

Occupation by Design Applications	Sensory Integration/NDT	Person-Environment-Occupation	Model of Human Occupation	Occupational Adaptation	Ecology of Human Performance
Appeal	The child's sensory integrative and neurodevelopmental abilities have a direct impact on the appeal of an occupation.	The unique characteristics of the child contribute to the appeal of an occupation for that child.	Appeal is demonstrated by the dynamic interaction of the child's volition, habituation, and performance capacity for participation in occupation. Appeal is subjective and shaped by individual child and family values and preferences.	Appeal is heavily emphasized in the following concepts: person, adaptive response, adaptation energy, adaptation response modes, and behaviors. The uniqueness of the occupation to a child and family is shaped through the understanding of these concepts.	The process of establishing or restoring skills occurs as a part of the occupational experience, while adaptations or modifications support participation in appealing occupations within natural contexts.
Intactness	The goodness of fit in the interaction between the child and the environment in which the occupation is occurring.	The environment (i.e., contexts and situations outside the child) is key to intactness.	Intactness is observed through the shaping of occupation by the physical and social elements within which it occurs. Engagement in occupation reflects rhythm, intensity, and duration in a particular environment. Opportunity is reflected in physical and social environments.	The environment is extremely powerful in this model as the desire for mastery blends the challenges of the occupation in the natural environment with the child.	Occupations in natural contexts support skill development or remediation, while adaptation of the environment/task or alteration of contextual dimensions (spatial/physical, temporal, and/or sociocultural) may support participation in occupation.

continued

Table 7-7 (continued)

AN INTEGRATIVE OVERVIEW ACROSS APPROACHES USING APPEAL, INTACTNESS, AND ACCURACY

Occupation by Design Applications	Sensory Integration/NDT	Person-Environment-Occupation	Model of Human Occupation	Occupational Adaptation	Ecology of Human Performance
Accuracy	Collaborative goal setting with the family considers the child's sensory and neurodevelopmental needs.	Occupational performance is a result of the match between the child, the environment, and the occupation.	Occupational participation, occupational performance, and skills all are viewed as important to accuracy. Participation and performance of occupations in natural environments best demonstrate the child's abilities.	Adaptation captures the creative problem solving exhibited by the child, the family, and the therapist. Evaluation of specific outcomes and responses to engagement in occupation helps to refine occupational performance in the natural context.	Anticipation of possible future occurrences is linked to collaborative goal setting in order to prevent negative outcomes, while collaborative goal setting and therapist design skills create opportunities for engagement in occupations based on individual or population needs.

Case Study: Janie

This case study example follows a young child, Janie, and her family over time as they negotiate the transition from early intervention services to preschool special education services, rise to the challenges of Janie's first year in preschool, and then transition again at age 5 to kindergarten. Janie's mother, Teresa, is a Spanish teacher in a local high school and her father, Miguel, is a manager of a local copy shop. While her parents are at work, Janie is cared for by Teresa's mother, Alma. Janie has a brother, Tomas, who is 3 years older. Throughout the case example, Janie and her family must collaborate with many professionals and work within different systems to ensure their needs are met. The occupational therapists change with the transitions. An overview of the therapy process will be provided through the lens of the Occupation by Design model and the different practice models utilized by each therapist.

Early Intervention

Eighteen-month-old Janie was diagnosed with developmental delays and referred to the state early intervention system. As part of a transdisciplinary approach to early intervention, Janie's parents could choose one professional to provide services while other disciplines would be considered consultants. During the initial early intervention team meeting, the Individualized Family Service Plan (IFSP) was developed and the team, which included Teresa and Miguel, decided to have occupational therapy be the lead service. It was also decided that therapy would occur in community settings, which included the home, playgroups, and the playground. Due to constraints in payment for early intervention services, occupational therapy could be provided no more than one time a week for an hour.

Lisa, the early intervention occupational therapist, was asked to provide services in part because she was bilingual and the family speaks only Spanish in the home. She began working with Janie shortly after the IFSP was finalized. At that time, Lisa noticed that Janie spent a lot of time with and stayed close by her mother and grandmother. Janie would maintain interest in activities her mother and grandmother were engaged in, but demonstrated limited interest in manipulating age-appropriate toys, did not touch or pick up food for self-feeding, and would become upset when they moved away from her, even if they were still within sight. Janie did not crawl, instead preferring to "scoot" her bottom on the floor by using her feet without touching her hands to the carpet.

On the IFSP, Teresa and Miguel had identified their main goals for Janie as: 1) Janie can feed herself finger foods, 2) Janie can crawl around the house, and 3) Janie will feel more confident to leave her mother and grandmother. During her first meeting with the family and Janie, Lisa reviewed the IFSP goals with the family. Lisa then performed an unstructured interview to obtain an occupational profile and determine more specific goals related to occupation. By beginning her session this way, Lisa was able to engage in the collaborative process of generating meaningful goals for Janie and her family as incorporated in Occupation by Design.

Three occupation-based goals were identified. The first was Janie will eat dinner with the family. Janie's parents told Lisa that Janie tended to prefer sitting on the floor next to her mother during dinner time and did not like to sit in her high chair. Her parents felt that eating meals as a family was important and wanted Janie to participate, particularly in eating the traditional Mexican foods that Alma often cooked. Lisa knew that she could work on self-feeding while still addressing the occupational experience of the family meal. The second goal was Janie will play in the tub when her father gives her a bath. Janie spent very little time alone with Miguel and did not like it when he participated in bath time, preferring her mother or grandmother instead. Teresa felt that bath time provided an opportunity for her to relax and it helped to share the family workload with Miguel. Lisa knew that by increasing the time Janie spent with her father, she could address the IFSP goal of Janie being more confident away from her mother and grandmother. The third occupation-based goal identified was Janie will play outside in the backyard. Janie disliked getting dirty or being in the grass. Since Janie's brother was an active 5-year-old, Teresa and Alma often took him outside to play. This created a problem because Janie would fuss and become upset. Lisa thought that she could simultaneously address crawling while working on playing outside.

Lisa had been an occupational therapist for 7 years and had worked in early intervention for 4 years. She had attended many continuing education workshops aimed specifically at pediatric practice. She was a member of a local group of occupational therapists who worked in pediatrics. They met monthly to discuss different interventions and the most recent research. Her experience and dedication to occupational therapy in early intervention gave her great ability to design creative and effective interventions, another aspect of accuracy that supported her work with Janie.

Over the next 12 months, Lisa provided therapy sessions one time a week for an hour. Sessions typically occurred around 5:00 p.m., timed so that all family members could participate. Dinner time and the beginning of bath time occurred in the early evening. Provision of therapy services with the participation of family members supported accuracy. The temporal context was taken into account by having sessions in the early evening; this supported intactness.

Lisa utilized a combination of the SI frame of reference and the EHP model as an approach to working with Janie and Janie's family. Lisa recognized that Janie's occupational performance was limited by sensory defensiveness, primarily overresponsivity to tactile input. Lisa taught Janie's parents to use activities that provided deep pressure and proprioceptive input in order to calm Janie. Lisa encouraged Janie's parents to put the couch cushions on the floor to provide a secluded play area and as a fun climbing structure as Janie became more confident with movement. Lisa showed Alma how to give deep pressure input to Janie's hands with a washcloth and then entice her to crawl across the living room rug. Lisa also coached Alma on how to do an oral motor program to decrease Janie's oral sensitivity prior to mealtimes and how to adapt traditional dishes to meet Janie's preferred tastes and textures. Lisa showed Teresa and Miguel how to swing Janie slowly in a blanket for calming before her bath. Janie's family learned how to combine sensory processing approaches with appealing occupations in order to support Janie's development.

Lisa knew, however, that a purely SI approach was not feasible in the natural context of the home. Instead, Lisa used the adapt/modify strategy from the EHP to further address Janie's sensory processing challenges. In order to ensure accuracy, Lisa collaborated with Janie's parents and grandmother to develop adaptations that would be a good fit with the family's routines: Janie's grandmother brought a large, fluffy blanket outside for Janie to sit on while playing, Janie's mother wedged stuffed animals in the high chair beside Janie to help her feel more secure during dinner time, and Miguel and Teresa began bathing Janie and Tomas together with Miguel spending more and more time alone with both children each night. Through collaboration and adaptation of the natural context, the interventions supported both accuracy and intactness.

PRESCHOOL

By the time Janie was 33 months old, she was walking, finger feeding, and spending time alone with her father without difficulty. The team had set new goals for Janie and

Lisa felt that Janie was in the process of meeting them. Janie still demonstrated general developmental delays, however, in motor, adaptive, and cognitive domains. When she turned 3 years old, Janie was to transition to the preschool program in the local school district where she would continue to receive occupational therapy services.

Lisa tried repeatedly, but without success, to contact the preschool's occupational therapist, Carrie, in order to discuss Janie's progress and provide recommendations. Lisa hoped to attend the transition meeting where the Individualized Education Program (IEP) was developed but was unable due to a scheduling conflict. Carrie did not feel that it was important to speak with Lisa. She appreciated knowing information about Janie's progress in early intervention, but believed she could get all the information she needed through a copy of the IFSP. The issues surrounding the two therapists' lack of communication resulted in a deficit in accuracy. The collaboration between therapists from each setting had the potential to provide a solid foundation for Janie as she transitioned into a new system.

Carrie had been an occupational therapist for almost 20 years. She had worked in the same preschool for 12 years and was well known in the community as an expert with young children who had special needs. She was also a frequent presenter at state meetings, typically providing information on preschool services. Carrie's high level of expertise and years of experience helped to support her ability to create highly accurate interventions.

Carrie met Janie's parents at the first IEP meeting. Carrie was asked to attend by the preschool special education teacher. Carrie listened to Teresa's and Miguel's concerns about Janie and their own anxieties about sending her to a preschool program. Janie had never participated in any programs outside of the home. In early intervention, Lisa had encouraged the family to begin weekly play groups with Janie in order to help prepare her to be around children her own age. Janie had begun to do well in these play groups, engaging with the other children for short periods of time before retreating back to her parents. Now Janie would be in a real classroom with 11 children, all 3 year olds. Both parents thought it might be best if Janie stayed at home and waited at least another year before entering school. Teresa was on the verge of tears as she expressed herself to Carrie.

Carrie had heard this from parents before. She understood the difficulty Janie's parents were experiencing. Carrie ascribed to the OA model. The entire transition process was made up of various occupational challenges for Janie and her family. She knew that the family was engaging in primitive response behaviors and that the transition process seemed overwhelming. In order to assist Janie's parents to demonstrate more mature adaptive response behaviors, Carrie first spent some time explaining how occupational therapy would work with Janie to help her adjust to the classroom. Carrie also suggested that Janie attend for short periods of time during the first few weeks. Carrie then took Teresa and Miguel on a tour of the classroom, showing them the various learning centers and asked them to provide some initial information regarding Janie's likes and dislikes. Teresa and Miguel left the preschool meeting feeling more positive about the transition. They began thinking of ideas for Carrie regarding classroom adaptations that might support Janie's needs. In addition to supporting a mature adaptive response from Janie's parents, Carrie was able to support accuracy in her interventions by spending time with them and gaining an idea of Janie's potential classroom requirements.

Three months into the school year, Janie was coming to school for the full morning session and beginning to engage with the other children in her class. The main areas of occupational therapy intervention were participation in play, socialization with peers, and performance of self-help skills. Through her use of the OA model, Carrie was able to determine how best to support Janie to participate in various classroom occupations.

For instance, Carrie noted that Janie was able to participate in center activities for short periods, but would become upset and stressed prior to the end of center time. The room was loud during centers, as the other children were typically roaming about and playing. Carrie recognized Janie's response as dysadaptive and met with the preschool teacher to determine possible options. They contacted Janie's parents by phone to obtain their input. Teresa explained how Janie often retreated to a small area in her closet when she was feeling stressed. Inside she had all her stuffed animals and blankets to cuddle.

Carrie and the teacher decided to add a large cardboard box to the corner of the classroom. All the children helped decorate the outside. Several pillows were placed in the inside and a curtain was attached over the opening. The box became the resting place for all the children in the classroom. Janie used it anytime she was feeling upset and needed a break. Carrie noticed that Janie frequently used the resting place during center time—staying in for a few minutes until she felt able to return to the rest of the class. Over time, Janie spent progressively more time participating in centers and less time in the resting place. Through this intervention, Carrie was supporting a more mature adaptive response from Janie while modifying the occupational environment, and simultaneously supporting a restorative occupation with great appeal.

KINDERGARTEN

After 2 years in the preschool program, Janie was ready to make the transition to kindergarten. Janie's parents met with Carrie and the rest of the team members to discuss transition needs. Elise, the kindergarten's occupational therapist, also attended the meeting. Carrie provided Elise with information about Janie's occupational functioning in the preschool classroom. She invited Elise to visit the classroom to observe Janie. Elise had a caseload of over 60 students, however, and was unable to find time to visit. During the meeting, Elise had to leave early to drive to another school in the county. She was unable to speak individually with Janie's parents. Accuracy was affected by this limited collaboration. Elise was unable to obtain information about Janie and did not know the parent's priorities for school-based therapy.

Elise had graduated the previous year with her degree in occupational therapy. She had worked in the school system for 1 year and had received some mentoring from a more experienced therapist in the district. With a large caseload, limited experience, and travel to eight schools, Elise was feeling overwhelmed. Her ability to create accurate interventions for her students was constrained by these factors.

Janie had made significant progress during preschool. She now had a "best friend," Debra, who she played with both in and out of class. Her increased engagement in art activities, such as finger painting, and eating a wider variety of food textures suggested improvements in sensory processing. Janie continued to have delays in motor skills, particularly gross motor, and this was especially evident on the playground. Janie often seemed "stuck" during recess, standing and staring at the other children but unsure how to proceed. This concerned Janie's parents and they were looking forward to addressing gross motor skills in kindergarten.

The school administrators, teachers, and Elise had different ideas. Janie's challenges were not considered to be educationally related, except for her adaptive skills and fine motor skills. Based on Janie's educational needs, Elise, with the support of the school administrators and teacher, decided to provide occupational therapy on a consultation basis only. Teresa and Miguel were disappointed, but did not feel that there was an option for more services.

Since Elise would be providing occupational therapy on a consult basis there was additional pressure for her to make her interventions as intact, accurate, and appealing as possible. She decided that any intervention would need to incorporate the entire population of children in the classroom and be performed regularly as part of the classroom routine. Elise had learned the MOHO in her occupational therapy education program and it was her primary model of practice. Using a MOHO approach, she began by observing Janie in the kindergarten classroom and during recess. She noted that Janie had a habit of standing on the sidelines, tending not to jump in and participate in gross motor play, particularly on the playground when there were many children. Her timidity appeared related to a poor sense of body awareness and decreased ability to imitate others in order to learn new motor skills. Elise felt that Janie had little personal capacity to participate in gross motor play, but that she appeared to have a desire to engage with the other children. Elise knew that by building on Janie's personal capacity she could increase her self-efficacy in gross motor play, which would further increase her volition.

Elise met with Janie's teacher and discussed some ideas. They decided that the most accurate and intact way to address Janie's gross motor play would be to separate the class into small groups. During recess, the groups would spend time at different areas of the playground for a set amount of time and then rotate to another area when the teacher blew her whistle. Elise would observe the class and help create the groups based on the children's gross motor abilities. Each group would have children with different skill levels. This would give Janie an opportunity to play on the equipment with only three or four other children. Elise gave the teacher ideas for how to assist Janie to initiate and engage in play. Elise also spoke with the physical education teacher and provided information about ways to support Janie.

Elise consulted on Janie one time a month during recess. Each time she observed Janie demonstrating increasingly more engagement on the playground equipment. She noticed that Janie appeared happy during recess and even initiated some play on her own. By playing in smaller groups, Janie was able to gain more control, practice her gross motor skills in a safe atmosphere, and increase her sense of personal causation. Although her gross motor skills were not at the same level as her peers, she was able to participate in an appealing occupation. Janie's volition supported her occupational engagement. She began to develop an interest in gross motor play, seeking out other girls in her class to make up games on the playground, and thus supporting her roles of friend and playmate.

Teresa and Miguel remained concerned about Janie's motor delays. Miguel's insurance would pay for 25 visits of outpatient occupational therapy per year, so they decided to start occupational therapy services at a private practice close to their home. Sara, the occupational therapist, had been in private practice for 15 years and had been an occupational therapist for 18 years. She had extensive continuing education and training in SI, but had recently become acquainted with the PEO model at a national meeting. Prior to learning about the PEO model, Sara provided therapy in her 900-square-foot SI gym. The gym contained steel beams with hooks that could hold many different types of swings. There was a large ball pit and a loft with a trapeze. Children who came to Sara's clinic loved therapy and their parents reported changes in their children's functioning. Yet, there continued to be problems with carry-over of skills to the home, school, and other community settings. After learning about the PEO model, Sara decided that her services would be more intact and accurate if they were provided in the natural settings of the child as well as the therapy gym.

Janie began occupational therapy with Sara once a week for an hour. For the first 3 months, Sara provided therapy in the gym with a focus on addressing Janie's motor planning skills and lingering sensory processing issues. Sara's experience in providing services supported her ability to design accurate interventions that were highly appealing to Janie, such as playing scavenger hunt in the ball pit, jumping from the trapeze onto a soft mattress, and picking up balls from the floor to throw at a target while swinging.

Based on her SI background, Sara believed that Janie's nervous system was changing and developing. Still, the interventions lacked the intactness needed to reinforce carry-over into the community.

As Janie became more confident with her skills, Sara suggested to Teresa and Miguel that therapy begin to take place in community settings. First, Sara met Janie and her parents at a local playground. Tomas was there as well. Sara taught the children some games to play on the playground equipment and gave Janie verbal cues to practice the motor movements needed to participate. After a few weeks of meeting on the playground, Sara went to Janie's home. In collaboration with Teresa and Miguel, Sara developed games and play activities that could be incorporated into Janie's day to assist in building her motor skills. Sara worked with Janie's parents to develop additional strategies for adapting the environment based on Janie's continuing sensory defensiveness. The strategies were also enmeshed within the family's daily routine in order to avoid disruption of current occupations. By using the top-down approach advocated by the PEO model, in conjunction with a bottom-up approach supported by SI, Sara was able to develop interventions that were contextually intact and bolstered Janie's abilities in all environments.

Case Study Learning Activity

1. Review Table 7-7 and identify the parts of the case example that relate to the various models and frames of reference.

2. For the various age periods, consider alternative models and problem solve potential approaches from different perspectives. Provide a rationale for your alternate choices.

3. Use one of the case examples from another chapter and discuss an alternative model for approaching the occupational concerns. Discuss appeal, intactness, and accuracy aspects. Provide examples of treatment strategies that would relate to the chosen model.

Recommendations for Future Practice and Research

This chapter provides a summary to this book's presentation of five approaches to family-centered occupational therapy through several steps: 1) reviewing the clinical reasoning processes of occupational therapists, 2) considering each approach within the broad perspective of Occupation by Design (Pierce, 2001, 2003), 3) comparing the approaches, and 4) providing a case that demonstrates the implementation of different approaches by different therapists as a child transitions from one phase of services to another. Each therapist will make use of these approaches in a different way, within the unique challenges of his or her daily practice.

POPULATION/CONSULTATIVE PERSPECTIVE

Population and consultative perspectives are critical components for exploration as we look to our future needs in providing occupational therapy services to infants, children, and their families. As noted in Chapter 1, we must secure our place at the table by using occupation-based models. Through our valuable focus on daily occupational performance, we will reinforce our domain of concern and the value of our expertise in providing services to this population. Occupation by Design offers a very broad clinical reasoning perspective, in order to help occupational therapists solidify and effectively apply their understanding of occupation. As noted in each of the chapters, we continue to need tools or media through which we provide specific interventions. Thus, the use of frames of reference and models will continue to serve us well in adapting occupations based on individual person, task, and contextual considerations. But, we must not allow ourselves to narrow our perspectives so much that we lose sight of the larger picture: the satisfaction of authentic occupations for infants, children, and their families.

Fostering engagement in occupation in the childhood population is an opportunity for occupational therapists to move beyond medically based practice and into community and social environments. The work we have done with infants and families has prepared us to move into population-based interventions. We have been innovative in recognizing the value of synthesizing multiple modes of clinical reasoning with this population to provide unique services. Our challenge is to effectively place authentic occupation and our knowledge of occupation at the center of our practice, as encouraged by Yerxa (1967). By addressing population-centered perspectives, multiple opportunities are available to occupational therapists. Consultation is an expected skill for use in any of the occupation-based models. Appreciation of, and scholarship in the use of, appeal, intactness, and accuracy are all central to our advanced participation in quality practice. We are at the forefront of change. Occupational therapists possess the expertise to lead this challenge. Let us incorporate and shape the future of pediatric practice through our continued commitment in the use and study of authentic occupation.

REALIZING OCCUPATIONAL THERAPY'S VISION OF FAMILY-CENTERED AND OCCUPATION-BASED PRACTICE: THREE BRIDGES TO CHANGE

As has been argued elsewhere by Pierce (2001), change toward increasingly occupation-based practice requires the building of three bridges: a generative discourse, demonstration projects, and education emphasizing occupation-based practice. These three bridges would also serve well to support the development of family-centered occupational therapy. A generative discourse in regard to family-centered services would identify and share with others in the profession a rich variety of new concepts, approaches, and tools that support family-centered care more effectively. Demonstration projects are centers that aspire to best practices. Opportunities to test and refine such practices in family-centered and occupation-based occupational therapy enrich the field through their discoveries and their modeling of innovative practice that is true to the principles of family-centeredness. Last of the three bridges is education that provides students with training in best practices of family-centered occupational therapy.

Given that not all occupational therapists are presently providing truly family-centered services, we might wonder how a generative discourse, demonstration sites, and education targeting best practice family-centered occupational therapy might be put in place? We recommend change methods to support such efforts, large or small. Change methods take many forms, but basically they recommend the following: selection by a small team of two or three practitioners of an important but doable improvement in their everyday practices, a trial of the improvement, reflection and discussion of the trial, refinement of the new procedure, and, if the team is pleased with the outcomes of the change, dissemination of the change to other small teams (Langley, Nolan, Nolan, Norman, & Provost, 1996; Stringer, 1999). Creative design process (Pierce, 2001, 2003) may also be of help in such efforts to make occupational therapy more family centered. Just imagine the kinds of changes that may support such services: changes in assessments, in the locations and contexts of intervention, in the degree of inclusion of the family in therapeutic interventions, or in the family friendliness of the clinical setting. Even the smallest change is valuable.

And of course, we cannot conclude this final chapter without the inevitable call for research. Research, research! We hunger always for greater understanding of the complex requirements of assisting children and families. Our profession and discipline is growing by leaps and bounds. Already some of our great researchers are at work, describing the challenges of family occupational patterns in the presence of a child with disability and studying the challenges of family-centered care. Let us show our appreciation of those who are already engaged in this valuable work, and let's hope their ranks are swelled further by dedicated researchers ready to contribute to our developing knowledge of the occupational patterns of families and children, the thinking of occupational therapists as they provide family-centered services, the development of tools and approaches to support that care, and studies of the outcomes of occupational therapy centered on the needs of infants, children, and families.

References

Clouder, L. (2000). Reflective practice: Realizing its potential. *Physiotherapy, 86,* 517-522.

Fleming, M. (1991). The therapist with the three-track mind. *American Journal of Occupational Therapy, 45,* 1007-1014.

Graham, I. W. (2000). Reflective practice and its role in mental health nurses' practice development: A year-long study. *Journal of Psychiatric and Mental Health Nursing, 7,* 109-117.

Hooper, B. (1997). The relationship between pretheoretical assumptions and clinical reasoning. *American Journal of Occupational Therapy, 51,* 328-338.

Javetz, R., & Katz, N. (1989). Knowledgeability of theories of occupational therapy practitioners in Israel. *American Journal of Occupational Therapy, 43,* 664-675.

Lagerlov, P., Loeb, M., Andrew, M., & Hjortdahl, P. (2000). Improving doctors' prescribing behavior through reflection on guidelines and prescription feedback. *Quality in Health Care, 9,* 159-165.

Langley, G. J., Nolan, K. M., Nolan, T. W., Norman, C. L., & Provost, L. P. (1996). *The improvement guide: A practical approach to enhancing organizational performance.* San Francisco: Jossey-Bass.

Mattingly, C. (1991). What is clinical reasoning? *American Journal of Occupational Therapy, 45,* 979-986.

Mattingly, C., & Fleming, M. (1994). *Clinical reasoning: Forms of inquiry in a therapeutic practice.* Philadelphia: F.A. Davis Co.

Neuhaus, B. E. (1988). Ethical considerations in clinical reasoning: The impact of technology and cost containment. *American Journal of Occupational Therapy, 42,* 288-294.

Paget, T. (2001). Reflective practice and clinical outcomes: Practitioners' views on how reflective practice has influenced their clinical practice. *Journal of Clinical Nursing, 10,* 204-214.

Pierce, D. (2001). Occupation by design: Dimension, therapeutic power, and creative process. *American Journal of Occupational Therapy, 55,* 249-259.

Pierce, D. (2003). *Occupation by design: Building therapeutic power.* Philadelphia: F.A. Davis Co.

Reilly, M. (1974). *Play as exploratory learning.* Beverly Hills, CA: Sage Publications.

Rogers, J. C. (1983). Eleanor Clark Slagle lectureship—1983. Clinical reasoning: The ethics, science and art. *American Journal of Occupational Therapy, 37,* 601-616.

Schell, B., & Cervero, R. (1993). Clinical reasoning in occupational therapy: An integrative review. *American Journal of Occupational Therapy, 47,* 605-610.

Schon, D. (1983). *The reflective practitioner: How professionals think in action.* New York: Basic Books.

Stringer, E. (1999). *Action research* (2nd ed.). Thousand Oaks, CA: Sage Publications.

Unsworth, C. (2005). Using head-mounted video camera to explore current conceptualizations of clinical reasoning in occupational therapy. *American Journal of Occupational Therapy, 59*(1), 31-40.

Ward, J. D. (2003). The nature of clinical reasoning with groups: A phenomenological study of an occupational therapist in community mental health. *American Journal of Occupational Therapy, 57,* 625-634.

Yerxa, E. J. (1967). Authentic occupational therapy: The 1966 Eleanor Clark Slagle lecture. *American Journal of Occupational Therapy, 21,* 1-9.

INDEX

WAIT
...*There's More!*

Best Practice Occupational Therapy: In Community Service with Children and Families
Winnie Dunn, PhD, OTR, FAOTA
400 pp., Soft Cover, 2000, ISBN 10: 1-55642-456-6, ISBN 13: 978-1-55642-456-4, Order# 34566, **$50.95**

This text applies theoretical and evidence-based knowledge to best practice with emphasis on children and families in community settings. It emphasizes best practice and incorporates clinical reasoning and practice models into the material. Students are provided with methods for working through the problem-solving processes as they learn the material.

Developmental and Functional Hand Grasps
Sandra J. Edwards, MA, OTR, FAOTA; Donna J. Buckland, MS, OTR; Jenna D. McCoy-Powlen, MS, OTR
128 pp., Soft Cover, 2002, ISBN 10: 1-55642-544-9, ISBN 13: 978-1-55642-544-8, Order# 35449, **$48.95**

This text is designed to identify, illustrate, and describe the complexity of grasps in a clear, user-friendly manner. Faculty, clinicians, and students will find that this accurate and comprehensive text addresses essential developmental, precision, and power grasps as well as handwriting grasps for use in evaluation, treatment, and research.

Quick Reference Dictionary for Occupational Therapy, Fourth Edition
Karen Jacobs, EdD, OTR/L, CPE, FAOTA; Laela Jacobs, OTR/L
600 pp., Soft Cover, 2004, ISBN 10: 1-55642-656-9, ISBN 13: 978-1-55642-656-8, Order# 36569, **$29.95**

Occupational Therapy: Performance, Participation, and Well-Being, Third Edition
Charles H. Christiansen, EdD, OTR, OT(C), FAOTA; Carolyn M. Baum, PhD, OTR/L, FAOTA; Julie Bass-Haugen, PhD, OTR/L, FAOTA
680 pp., Hard Cover, 2005, ISBN 10: 1-55642-530-9, ISBN 13: 978-1-55642-530-1, Order# 35309, **$69.95**

OT Study Cards in a Box, Second Edition
Karen Sladyk, PhD, OTR/L, FAOTA
255 Cards w/Carrier, 2003, ISBN 10: 1-55642-620-8, ISBN 13: 978-1-55642-620-9, Order# 36208, **$46.95**

Understanding and Managing Vision Deficits: A Guide for Occupational Therapists, Second Edition
Mitchell Scheiman, OD
400 pp., Soft Cover, 2002, ISBN 10: 1-55642-528-7, ISBN 13: 978-1-55642-528-8, Order# 35287, **$42.95**

Documentation Manual for Writing SOAP Notes in Occupational Therapy, Second Edition
Sherry Borcherding, MA, OTR/L
256 pp., Soft Cover, 2005, ISBN 10: 1-55642-719-0, ISBN 13: 978-1-55642-719-0, Order# 37190, **$35.95**

Measuring Occupational Performance: Supporting Best Practice in Occupational Therapy, Second Edition
Mary Law, PhD, OT Reg. (Ont.), FCAOT; Carolyn Baum, PhD, OTR/C, FAOTA; Winnie Dunn, PhD, OTR, FAOTA
440 pp., Hard Cover, 2005, ISBN 10: 1-55642-683-6, ISBN 13: 978-1-55642-683-4, Order# 36836, **$48.95**

Vision, Perception, and Cognition: A Manual for the Evaluation and Treatment of the Adult with Acquired Brain Injury, Fourth Edition
Barbara Zoltan, MA, OTR/L
368 pp., Hard Cover, 2007, ISBN 10: 1-55642-738-7, ISBN 13: 978-1-55642-738-1, Order# 37387, **$44.95**

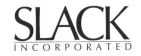